UNFILTERED REDUX

Exploring uncharted depths of mind:
where masks fall and wisdom emerges

Dr. Patricia A. Farrell

ISBN: 979-8-9930004-2-8

BOOKS by Patricia A. Farrell, Ph.D. (may be purchased on a number of platforms, not limited to Amazon)

When You Can't Pour From an Empty Glass: CBT Skills for Exhausted Caregivers

The Little Book on Learning Big Critical Thinking Skills

Unfiltered: Beneath the noise of our thoughts lies the true narrative of our minds. An honest journey into psychology when the masks finally come off.

Unfiltered Again: A behind-the-scenes look at healthcare, medicine and mental health

How to Be Your Own Therapist: A Step-by-Step Guide to Taking Back Your Life

It's Not All in Your Head: Anxiety, Depression, Mood Swings & Multiple Sclerosis

Work Stress: How You Can Beat It

A Social Security Disability Psychological Claims Handbook

A Social Security Disability Psychological Claims Guidebook for Children's Benefits

The Disability Accessible US Parks in All 50 States: A Comprehensive Guide

UNFILTERED REDUX

Birding in the US NOW!: A birding guide for individuals with disabilities

Sleep, Insomnia, Stress:: What you don't know can hurt you

<u>Flash Fiction</u>

Unexpected Short Tales of Surprise

Contents

Introduction   1

Chapter 1: STOP! Brushing Your Teeth May Expose   5
You to DeadlyNeurotoxins

Chapter 2: Dismissing Cursive Is Like Throwing the   11
Baby Out with the Bathwater

Chapter 3: How to Win a War Without Weapons   15

Chapter 4: VIP Syndrome   19

Chapter 5: Spotlighting Emerging Dementia in Its   23
Many Iterations and Stages

Chapter 6: Headaches That Resist Treatment and the   29
Desperate Attempts to Crush Them

Chapter 7: When Is Exercise Not Exercise, and Is That   35
Good Enough?

Chapter 8: Psychotherapy That Is Pseudoscience Ac-   39
cording to Professionals: Conversion Therapy

Chapter 9: Rapunzel Wasn't Simply in a Castle; It's a   45
Psychiatric Syndrome

Chapter 10: Kindness and Charity Benefit Us More   49
Than We Know

Chapter 11: Cancer or Cognition: Where Does Nicotine Lie and Why the Controversy?   53

Chapter 12: Medical Devices Are Under Cyberattacks, and Your Life Could Be at Risk   57

Chapter 13: Doing Nothing, Including No 10K Steps, Is Good for Mental Health   60

Chapter 14: Exercise in Outdoor Greenery Has an Important Effect on MH and Brain   63

Chapter 15: Are You Writing in Cursive or On a Computer? It may make a difference in your creativity. What do/did the "greats" use?   68

Chapter 16: The Mind and Body May Respond to Acupuncture, Which Appears to Be Effective   73

Chapter 17: Skinnier, Sicker? Weight-Loss Meds' Raise Concerns   77

Chapter 18: Who Needs Homework or Education, Anyway?   81

Chapter 19: Where Have All the Sidewalks Gone?   87

Chapter 20: Death and the Cancer Screen Not Performed   91

Chapter 21: Public Places and Private Spaces   95

Chapter 22: Recipe for Creating Monsters   100

Chapter 23: The Nose May Determine Why Your Cognition Declines   106

Chapter 24: Stress Is the Brain Drain Robbing You of Everything   111

Chapter 25: Beware of the Hidden Mental Health Threats in Your Food   116

Chapter 26: Beyond Stereotypes: The Exceptional Abilities That Make Autistic Minds Invaluable   122

Chapter 27: Young Boys, Societal Shifting, Violence, and New Mental Health Concerns   129

Chapter 28: Understanding Sundowning: A Brief Guide for Families and Caregivers   140

Chapter 29: Not Just Another Day in May 1970   147

Chapter 30: A Reflex to Damage   150

Chapter 31: Pedophiles Are the Nicest People   154

Chapter 32: Mammo Silence   158

Chapter 33: No One Listens   161

Chapter 34: Transport Yourself Into Your Family's Future   167

Chapter 35: The New College Grind Isn't the Classes   170

Chapter 36: The Art of the Hidden Message   174

Chapter 37: One Shining Light Is Out: Mike Nichols   177

Chapter 38: Cosby: Another Icon Crumbling?   180

Chapter 39: Psychologists Guided Torture for CIA   183

Chapter 40: Psychologists Guided Torture for CIA   188

Chapter 41: Digitally Illiterate But Able to Learn   193

Chapter 42: A Lesson From The Joan Rivers Playbook   197

Chapter 43: Just a Pen, Not a Payment   200

Chapter 44: Brain Cleaning? Is That Something We Should Be Doing?   204

Chapter 45: Simple Isometric Exercises to Build Strength and Mental Wellness for All Ages   208

Chapter 46: Why Scientists Want You to Use Your Other Hand   213

Chapter 47: A Simple Touch Technique That's Backed by Multiple Studies   218

Chapter 48: The Productive and Powerful "Crumb Method" of Writing Creatively and Smart   224

Chapter 49: For I Was Hungry, and You Gave Me Food: Food insecurity and AI's hope for the future   228

Chapter 50: Monday, Monday, Anxiety Strikes and Sticks for a Lifetime   235

Chapter 51: The Science Is In: Your Dog/Cat Is Literally Saving Your Life   243

Chapter 52: Music Literally Rewires Your Brain and Heals Your Soul   247

Chapter 53:Do You Know the Many Forms of Dementia?   252

Chapter 54: Obesity Isn't a Simple Matter of Diet and Exercise — It's More Complex   258

Chapter 55: Digital Friends Offer Companionship to Lonely Kids   264

Chapter 56: Is the Air You Breathe Quietly Fueling Dementia?   270

Chapter 57: Timing When You Eat May Be the Secret to   274
Better Health

Chapter 58: CTE: The Hidden Danger Threatening   280
Athletes of All Ages

Chapter 59: The Algorithm That Gave Me Pause   287
Tonight and "Hooked" Me

Chapter 60: Startling Finding COVID-19 Caused   291
Cognitive Decline and Brain Aging?

Chapter 61: Your Body Has Its Own Clock — And It   296
Could Save Your Life

Chapter 62: Mental Health Secrets Are Being Unrav-   303
eled, and Inflammation Is the Culprit

Chapter 63: Starvation and Protein Restriction in Kids   313
Kills Bodies and Minds

Chapter 64: The Hidden Dangers of Mental Health   319
Chatbots: Why We Need to Act Now

Chapter 65: The Japanese Walking Secret That's   324
Changing Lives: How 30 Minutes Can Transform Your
Health

Chapter 66: Mental Health Secrets Are Being Unrav-   330
eled, and Inflammation Is the Culprit

Chapter 67: Pain Perception May Be Related to Your   339
Eye Coloring

Chapter 68: And Then There Was a NEW Personality   346
"Disorder" for Pondering

Chapter 69: The Height Problem No One Wants to   353
Talk About

Chapter 70: Surprise! Your Aging Brain Isn't Wearing   360
Thin — It's Retrofitting Its Layers

About the Author   365

Books by Dr. Patricia A. Farrell   367

A Special Request   369

Introduction

The current era of social media presentation requires the presentation of perfect images and sanitized news, while algorithms create echo chambers that make authentic voices difficult to find. Society today operates with condensed truths that replace complex information while it favors popularity over detailed explanations, and most critical dialogues occur in quiet conversations instead of prominent headlines. The purpose of "Unfiltered Redux" is to provide genuine information because modern society needs authentic insights that traditional discourse cannot deliver.

The third release of "Unfiltered" presents psychological realities that could surprise readers as well as challenge them and potentially cause disturbance. Throughout my decades as a licensed psychologist who worked with Alzheimer's patients at Mount Sinai Medical Center and Social Security Disability claimants, I observed how mental health descriptions in public discourse differ from actual real-world experiences.

These essays emerged from an unorthodox hypothesis that we should eliminate the practice of avoiding important subjects. We need to recognize that several urgent contemporary issues, including hidden threats in common products and psychological manipulation in digital environments, need more than shallow statements and political correctness.

The following pages reveal several unpalatable realities that typical media outlets choose to disregard. Neurotoxins exist in toothpaste products, which has been documented by science for the past fifty years. Young men face an unprecedented mental health emergency because of the manosphere's growing influence. Your Monday anxiety causes biological changes in your body that last for weeks despite being a mental condition.

The statements presented are evidence-based and derived from the author's extensive experience studying human behavior and societal patterns throughout his / her / their career. The chapters in "**Un-filtered Redux**" present crucial subjects that need honest analysis, including how doing nothing provides benefits and ultra-processed foods present secret mental health risks.

This book offers solutions beyond what standard self-help books provide, even though it focuses on problems. The book presents straightforward isometric exercises, which enhance both physical and mental health, along with scientific explanations about hand preference and musical effects on brain development and emotional healing. The book presents concrete strategies for managing dementia-related sundowning symptoms and the productive, creative writing approach known as the **Crumb Method**.

This collection stands out because it enters domains that many authors typically stay away from. The book analyzes how entertainment contains secret messages, discusses the increasing vulnerability of young boys to violent ideologies, and presents multiple studies that support touch techniques for healing. We will investigate the unpalatable aspects of healthcare systems together with education and social structures, which determine our daily existence.

The content of specific chapters might present challenges to particular readers or trigger controversy among them. That's intentional. Growth occurs when we challenge our comfort zones, while understanding emerges from studying subjects that most people prefer to ignore. The discussions about concealed pedophiles and brain-draining stress matter precisely because they represent difficult subjects.

The book presents findings from over thirty years of clinical work and research alongside real-world experience that provide actionable knowledge for modern life navigation. Readers who seek more than surface-level thinking guidance about their world will benefit from this book.

The book "Unfiltered Redux" provides no simple solutions or comforting realities. Through its pages, readers gain essential abilities to detect illusions while discovering the fundamental mechanisms that influence both personal and social experiences. The book belongs to those who accept challenging realities rather than those who want pleasant deceptions in our split society between comfort-seekers and truth-seekers.

Are you prepared to uncover what exists beyond what meets the eye?

Chapter 1: STOP! Brushing Your Teeth May Expose You to DeadlyNeurotoxins

Are you sure the toothpaste you're using is safe and won't expose you or your kids to harm?

Emphasis on brushing our teeth has always been a central concern for those in dental healthcare, and both dentists and dental hygienists have demonstrated how to brush and what to use. But as far back as 1974, concerns about the dentifrices that we use were expressed in dental research publications.

At that time, surface enamel had a high lead content. A number of widely used dentifrices were tested for lead since it was suspected that they could be a source of this element. Every single sample tested positive for lead.

Toothpaste samples taken from certain brands showed high levels of lead in the areas immediately surrounding the product container's walls. When squeezed from nearly empty tubes, the paste contained substantial levels of lead in these tests. These findings left little doubt that these products contained a neurotoxin that could cause harm if ingested. How many years ago was that? Yes, that was 45 years ago, and we still use products that may not be safe. But what's the specific problem, and shouldn't we have been protected by the agencies given that charge?

Children and Lead Exposure

There are several well-documented negative impacts of lead exposure on children's health, including:

Brain and neurological system injury

Decreased development

Issues with learning and conduct disorders

Speech and hearing impairments

Resulting in:

Reduced intelligence of a lifelong nature

Minimal capacity for sustained attention

Academic underachievement

In children, we need to be especially concerned, as the brain is where the most damage can occur, and the consequences can be lifelong. Lead is harmful to children because it enters the bloodstream rapidly. The bloodstream transports lead to the brain, bones, and every part of a child's body. It is insidious and may not be detected immediately except when specific blood tests are performed. The question here, of course, is whether or not lead is suspected to be the culprit and testing is ordered.

A child's blood lead level will increase if they ingest lead. However, blood lead levels decline over time when a child's exposure to lead ends. However, despite decreasing levels of lead, not all lead will be eliminated, and this is where the damage lies.

Kidney, perspiration, and feces are excreted by the body as a portion of the lead. Bones are another repository for lead. Lead levels in bones can decline over decades. But there's more here than we would suspect, and we would be lulled into a false sense of security that the body has a natural ability to read itself of lead. The story is more complex than that.

Due to its ability to penetrate and remain in the body, lead is extremely harmful to children's health. Lead can enter the blood circulation and even reach the brain when a kid breathes lead dust or consumes lead particles. Remember the toothpaste that we mentioned earlier? Lead, alarmingly, can lodge in bones and soft tissues, where it can stay for decades, unlike many poisons that the body removes.

One reason lead is so harmful is that it resembles calcium and iron, two essential minerals necessary for a growing body. Lead, when ingested, mimics these essential nutrients and fools cells into utilizing them instead. This change disrupts the brain's normal development and functioning.

Like insulation, the protective myelin layer around nerve cells is likewise damaged by lead. Damage to this coating prevents the normal transmission of nerve signals throughout the brain. Physical and mental development, as well as learning and processing information, are all impacted by this harm. It is crucial to limit lead exposure in youngsters because the consequences can be long-lasting and happen at very low exposure levels.

Toothpaste Current Research

After all these years, researchers decided to revisit the exploration of currently available toothpastes and other potential sources of metal contamination. The results are anything but heartening and have raised new concerns for even the most well-known brands of toothpaste.

Many of the popular brands were included in a 2025 research project, and a chart is available here. In fact, you can find information on multiple products and their safety regarding contamination by lead or other materials here. It's not only toothpaste that we need to be concerned about because we've recently been made aware of contaminants, such as metals, in baby food.

In the area of toothpaste, especially for children, 51 brands were tested, and, unfortunately, even those that were supposed to be "green" had issues with contamination. Lead was present in approximately 90% of toothpastes, arsenic in 65%, mercury in slightly less than half, and cadmium in one-third. Many brands have some harmful substances. Many popular brands were found to contain harmful substances, including Crest, Sensodyne, Tom's of Maine, Dr. Bronner's, and others.

In their defense, several corporations have pointed out that lead is ubiquitous in nature and thus impossible to eliminate. Currently, the federal Baby Food Safety Act of 2024 is stuck in Congress, which would limit lead levels in children's food to 10 parts per billion. The lead limit in infant food in California is six parts per billion; however, this does not apply to toothpaste. The majority of toothpastes surpassed those levels.

You can find arsenic in nature just about everywhere: rocks, dirt, water, air, and even some living things. Organic chemicals, including those found in seafood (such as fish and shellfish), are one possible form they can take. However, when we detect unacceptable levels of any heavy metal, such as lead, in a product intended for oral use or ingestion, it is mandatory that we take every possible step to eliminate it. To do less is unconscionable and damaging to children and adults.

As always, it is wise to inform yourself about all the foods and materials that you will either ingest or apply to your body. This research would not have seemed necessary, except that almost 50 years ago, lead was found in toothpaste. Now that we have the information, we can act intelligently with it and protect ourselves and our children.

Chapter 2: Dismissing Cursive Is Like Throwing the Baby Out with the Bathwater

Computers have many advantages, but there are several that cursive handwriting has over them, and we need to pay attention to them.

In an era where technological advancements and digital communication predominate, cursive writing's value may seem to have diminished. Many contend that teaching cursive is an antiquated practice that is no longer necessary in the contemporary world. But it would be like throwing out the baby with the bathwater to completely disregard cursive handwriting instruction. Cursive writing offers numerous scholastic and cognitive benefits that warrant consideration.

Particularly in the early years of a child's schooling, cursive writing is crucial for cognitive development. Fine motor skills and hand-eye coordination, which are crucial for brain development, are needed to learn how to write in cursive. Students improve their dexterity and fortify the neurological connections between their brain and muscles as they practice writing in cursive. This active participation benefits reading, math, and other academic subjects in addition to writing.

Moreover, writing in cursive encourages improved information processing and memory retention. Writing in cursive simultaneously stimulates several brain areas, leading to a deeper comprehension of the material being written. Research shows that students who write notes in cursive do better than those who type. Better learning outcomes and critical thinking abilities are a result of this cognitive engagement.

Cursive is also beneficial in terms of motor skills and brain development. Brain imaging studies have shown that cursive is involved in a robust network that is supported by writing by hand rather than using a keyboard. The negative implications of abandoning cursive have been addressed by the National Institute of Health.

Research supported by the NIH has noted that "...*cursive writing has been considered an essential precursor for further academic success..., and the skill is typically acquired during childhood in societies with a strong literacy tradition.*" The fine finger movements of cursive carry much more importance than key clicking in terms of a wealth of benefits not fully understood at present.

If we studied cursive more, we would see how finger strength on the writing tool connects to the hand, which connects to the wrist. The wrist enables the hand to rotate while writing letters and numbers.

We understand that an aspect of integration reinforces both muscle movement and the brain's learning capacity. Making circles on lined paper is a good use of time and not a waste. Unfortunately, in our digital age, we often overlook the importance of cursive writing in education. This is not only a shame; it is a disservice to all of the students who will come to all of the schools where cursive is now seen as a useless activity.

Cursive writing also has cultural and historical significance. Students who master cursive have access to literature, handwritten letters, and historical documents in their original form. This link to the past not only deepens their awareness of history and culture but also fosters a love of the written word. We must preserve this cultural heritage as it demonstrates the evolution of human communication.

The act of using cursive also encourages creativity and self-expression. Contrary to the homogeneity of typed text, cursive enables people to add their own distinctive style to their handwriting. This personal touch makes written communication more appealing and inspires pupils to take pride in their penmanship. A sense of ownership over their writing might also enhance creativity and self-esteem.

In addition, the fluidity of cursive writing encourages better letter recognition and reading fluency. It aids children in comprehending the relationships between letters, words, and phrases, which is essential for proficient reading and writing. Discontinuing cursive would potentially impede language growth.

If anything is essential in early schooling, it is cursive. Handwriting instruction has numerous educational and brain-developmental benefits, as research over the past several decades has shown; ignoring it would be a regrettable mistake. Cursive writing is essential to a well-rounded education since it fosters creativity and preserves cultural heritage while also improving fine motor skills and cognitive engagement. We shouldn't undervalue the lasting value of this skill because it continues to mold students' minds and enhance their educational opportunities.

Chapter 3: How to Win a War Without Weapons

No one needs major firepower, supersonic aircraft or mountains of munitions to win a war. Of course, I mean not only wars in distant countries but also the wars that too many people are trying to win with armaments or hatred right here within the United States. Agreed, that means just about every war that is now ongoing around the world, but the two most virulent of wars are the ones that are centered around religious beliefs and ethnic superiority or white privilege, as it is currently being called.

"White privilege" is the latest buzzword that is setting off the media motormouths and firing up the talk shows that pull in their many "expert" consultants. White privilege is seen all around the world, and those who do not fit into this group are marginalized, left without work, education or the hope for a future. We see it right here in the United States.

Forget the fact that the media consultants do not really specialize in the actual topic of white privilege, but that seems to be irrelevant to the producers. They still, in fact, get psychologists and psychiatrists mixed up no matter how many times we try to help them see the big distinction: prescription pad, no prescription pad, basically.

They also schedule professionals who specialize in substance abuse disorders to talk about ethnic hatred. Far-fetched? I think so. We do not have those wonderful Johnny Carson "Carnac the Magnificent" hats that give us special powers to read the contents of sealed envelopes. Let's assume that we possess superpowers and proceed accordingly. Some people actually believe psychologists and psychiatrists know everything and can speak knowledgeably about any topic. One word here? Rubbish.

Why didn't we abandon the notion that we should fight wars with guns and that only bloodshed can bring about peace? How many bodies do we need to count in order to come to some agreement that it's enough to be called a victory? Or do we just keep on throwing more money into our defense budgets to pay for planes that don't fly and tanks that can't do what we thought they could, and just keep throwing good people onto the barricades to suffer and die or come home terribly wounded both mentally and physically?

Then, who pays the bills for all that carnage? You and I are asked to contribute to the many charitable causes to help these people who have been all but abandoned in their hour of need by the very politicians who cravenly sent them to fight. And let's not forget the graft we pay to politicians (in the form of legal goodies), governments who are our "friends," and the support we give to drug producers and the homes we buy for those without morals and who will lend a hand at a price. It's open-checkbook diplomacy, and I don't believe it's a state secret.

How do we win the two wars I mentioned previously? These are not wars requiring weapons, not if you consider words and dialog weapons. Where are those in government who haven't been corrupted by the lobbyists and who see that talking to each other, working together and helping bring about better understanding and respect for religious and cultural differences can be a potent "weapon?"

We have no quarrel with anyone who is Muslim or Jewish or Hindu or Buddhist or Christian. These are all religions built on the concepts of goodness, forgiveness, charity, and love. They have contributed mightily to the world culture we have come to know and about which too many are still ignorant. Read who the prophets are in all these religions and what they preached, and the distortions currently being foisted around now become so much drek. Read some of the literature of the Middle Ages and the situation between the Christians and the Muslims in Spain. Read what the great religious intellectuals of their time said about living together in this world with others.

Words are the way to peace, but too many petty men and women don't want to take that road because it denies them the adventure of gaining power from fear. They would oppress anyone who did not think as they did. It's a horrible repeat of something we've seen over the centuries and just another example of the venality that is so prevalent right now.

Psychologists over the years have run dozens of experiments showing how to get people to work together, even those who are at odds with each other, when danger presents itself. Read Sherif et al. classic Robber's Cave and then read more. The answers are there, but we refuse to use them.

You could read some works on brainwashing, too, because that seems to be in evidence these days. Political thought control is in full swing right now as presidential aspirations poke through, and sometimes I feel as though I'm living in a prison. What happens in prison? The prisoners are controlled by keeping the various groups fighting against each other so they can never launch a concerted effort for change to the prison. Sounds like politics, doesn't it?

Even the world leaders' march in Paris recently has been seen as disingenuous. Those in the front line have not been proponents of a free press and have jailed or tried to intimidate those who wish for an intelligent dialog between parties. It suits their needs, not those of the rest of us. Bombs and firepower have been their answer to dissent, as secret prisons and torture have been ours. It is not a proud history that we have written. When the real history books are written 20 years from now, there will be many horrified readers, but will they see the need to work for change? Or will the same old venality persist? Money, fame and power are more tantalizing than the mythical snake that tempted Eve in the Garden of Eden.

Do we need guns and explosives? Evil people do it because their purpose is to gain incredible power through brutality, but peace and religious understanding? No, that's not for them. They don't even understand their own religion and the writing of the prophets, but they use religion as their standard. No, I don't believe those involved in the Inquisition were good, religious people, either. They got power through torture, didn't they?

When true intellect proves dangerous to a power play, intellect is refuted as the work of some dark force to be whipped out. How do they do it? Of course, children must be blown up in marketplaces and whole towns slaughtered. The media stands silently by in many instances, as they have in Africa. They don't even try to use words.

Chapter 4: VIP Syndrome

Famous people receive superior medical care, don't they? Popular belief supports this myth, despite instances where it is glaringly apparent that being a VIP may actually prevent you from receiving the usual standard of care. Usual? Should a VIP receive the usual standard of care or something above it? Ah, there lies the rub.

The "VIP Syndrome" has been a term kicking around in the medical literature since about 1964, when someone first noticed that being a celebrity could cause harm in a medical setting. Whenever a procedure is to be performed or a test initiated, there is a standard manner in which it is to be handled, but knowing that you're working on a celebrity changes the whole scenario. How could it not?

Psychological factors enter every medical setting just as they enter all other aspects of our lives, and people in healthcare are just as prone to its influences as we, somewhat infamous, mortals. In fact, we might end up getting better care because the usual standard of care is practiced, not care that is affected by factors such as concern for mistakes, press reactions, sudden media interest in the procedure or the person performing it, etc. How burdensome is that? Well, it surely doesn't make it easier for the famous patient, either, although they think they're getting platinum-level care in a luxury setting and with stellar doctors.

Media stories about famous patients abound and you just have to Google *Maurice Gibb, Andy Warhol, Joan Rivers, Queen Frederika of Greece, Mario Lanza*, and others to get some idea that being famous may not be such a good thing when it comes to healthcare.

Oh, and despite what the recent *Ken Burns* special on the Roosevelts indicated, a medical journal article attributes *Eleanor Roosevelt's* death to celebrity as well. Now that years have passed since her death, her medical records have been unsealed.

She was misdiagnosed, according to new reports, and she did not have the aplastic anemia reported in the documentary. The actual illness was tuberculosis involving the bone marrow. Her physician was a very close friend. She lived with him and his wife. In healthcare, this type of dual relationship is frowned on because it can cloud clinical judgment.

So, what happens here that puts these VIPs at greater risk? Simply put, it's a willingness to bend the rules, according to one article in the medical literature. The article goes on to provide nine principles for caring for these special patients.

The Nine Principles of Care for VIPs

1. Don't bend the rules. The standard of care for everyone must be strictly adhered to, even in the case of famous patients.

2. Work as a team. Everyone involved in the procedures must know who the primary medical person is and be totally familiar with all aspects of the disorder or procedure.

3. Communication is central. Again, everyone must be involved in these closely coordinated cases, and there must be a free flow of in-

formation between the patient and all involved healthcare personnel, plus security personnel.

4. Media communication must be carefully managed via a specific and planned media strategy.

5. Avoid "Chairmanship Syndrome," where the patient or the family believes that the chair of the department is the most appropriate person to handle the treatment. This may not be the case.

6. Care should be provided where it is most appropriate. This is especially important when intensive care is called for and luxury suites or amenities do nothing to improve the care at that point. Later, this can relieve the stress of the VIP, but not at the crucial time for intensive care.

7. Security is extremely important, more so in the case of VIPs because of the temptations associated with revealing information. We saw this in the case of *George Clooney*'s motorcycle accident in NJ.

8. Gifts can prove to be a problem. This can cause misunderstandings during the period of care as well as afterward.

9. Special care must be taken when working with the VIP's personal physician and any outside personnel they wish to bring in for consultation. In NYC, when a particular member of royalty seeks treatment at a major hospital, the entire floor on which he is seen is taken by him, his security and his entourage. This alone can present problems with other patients who must be moved.

How many medical professionals follow these nine simple rules? Not all of them, it would seem.

Chapter 5: Spotlighting Emerging Dementia in Its Many Iterations and Stages

Dementia's devastation may slip under our notice unless we recognize its many manifestations in behavior, speech, and mood.

The neatly dressed, immaculately groomed, and coiffed woman sat before me with a pleasant smile. She wore stylish, designer eyeglasses and looked at me like I were someone she recognized, but we had never met. For a moment, she hesitated, took off her glasses, and put them down on the table between us.

Now, the challenge was to assess her dementia level, how it affected her life, and if a new clinical trial medication might help. Part of the protocol required that she read something, and other parts required that she perform an action or recall items shown to her, and she would need her glasses for these tests.

She stared at her glasses as if they were odd objects and didn't know what to do with them. Turning the glasses over and examining them, she still didn't understand what they were meant to do.

Her daughter, who accompanied her for the evaluation, was almost in tears as she told me, "It has become even worse when we sit down for dinner because she doesn't know what is food and what utensils are. She often tries to eat her fork, and we have to stop her."

The woman was in her early 70s and previously had a successful clothing design business. But there had been noticeable slips in her behavior and even her ability to keep her company's accounts correct. A math whiz, she kept blaming it on the sunlight coming in through the windows in her office.

She no longer went to the office after daily arguments, and her suspicion regarding her staff disrupted her business. Previously, she enjoyed good interactions with everyone in the office. Most had worked with her for decades and were shocked at her behavior.

The Thief We Fail to Acknowledge

Dementia prevalence increases in direct correlation with age; it reaches 1% in the 60–64 age group and 24–33% in the 85+ age group. The term "dementia with late onset" refers to the disorder's emergence after the age of 65, whereas "early-onset dementia" describes its incidence before that age. The signs may be subtle, and even experienced clinicians may miss the probable diagnosis of dementia.

Roughly half of the 600 older persons whose brain scans and health indicators were investigated went on to acquire cognitive impairment.

In addition to signs of brain aging, they found that the genotype, specific cognitive test scores, hearing loss, memory problems reported by the individual themselves, and symptoms of depression were associated with future cognitive impairment in older individuals who were otherwise neurologically healthy.

According to a recent study, people with dementia start losing weight at least ten years before their symptoms appear, and this process speeds up in the two to four years leading up to the diagnosis. Dementia progression may be accelerated by hormonal and metabolic changes associated with weight reduction.

I can remember a neighbor who lived alone, was in her 80s, and went out several times a week to volunteer with, as she said," the elderly at the local hospital." No, she never saw herself as elderly or incapable of caring for all of her needs.

But one day, she mentioned to me that she had an evil twin coming into her home and hiding things on her. "I know she's hiding things," she said, "because I find them in places I would never have put them." It was at this point that she stopped preparing food for herself, and I had to arrange for a local senior-support organization to deliver meals to her. But things got worse, and she was becoming more mentally unstable until she was evaluated by a healthcare professional from that local hospital.

Once the evaluation was completed and she went to meet a team that worked on a dementia-related unit at the hospital where she had volunteered, she related the story of the evil twin. The decision was made that she could be admitted, and they would care for her.

Within months of arriving on the unit, she was discovered to have advanced cancer, had three surgeries, and died. We will never know if her dementia was related, somehow, to her cancer or the use of pain medication for it.

What Do We Look For?

Some of the subtle and not so subtle changes that should be noted in potential neurocognitive changes:

Losing track of newly acquired knowledge. Another symptom is an increase in the frequency with which you need to use memory aides, as well as a tendency to forget crucial dates or events.

Difficulty maintaining track of regular expenses or following a tried-and-true recipe.

Navigating to a known place, problems with a shopping list, or recalling the rules of a beloved game.

Sometimes they need assistance with the microwave's settings or recording a TV program.

Perplexed by events that do not unfold in real time. They could become disoriented and lose track of their way at times.

Has problems maintaining balance or reading. They might also have trouble seeing colors or gauging contrast, which could make them a dangerous driver.

Difficulty keeping up with or contributing to a discussion. They might repeat themselves or freeze up in the midst of a sentence, leaving you to figure out what to say next. They might not know how to spell certain words, have problems identifying commonplace objects, or even call something the wrong name (such as a "watch" being called a "hand-clock"). One thing to remember is that sometimes there are regional names for certain things, such as a door knocker may be called something else.

Possibly misplace items and not be able to trace their path back to them. As the illness advances, he or she may begin to falsely accuse others of stealing.

Perhaps they are careless with their money or do not keep themselves clean. Lack of care for personal cleanliness can also be caused by depression.

Do not participate in extracurricular activities, hobbies, or social gatherings. If they have a favorite team or pastime, they could struggle to keep up. And feelings of bewilderment, suspicion, depression, anxiety, or terror may set in. Whether they are at home, with friends, or somewhere else, they could quickly become agitated.

Although there are numerous changes that we may notice, there are a number of other reasons that some of these changes may be due to something else. We know that medication as well as a loss of active involvement in work or some other activity may be the reason for changes in behavior.

Remember, don't jump to a conclusion that the person is suffering from a cognitive impairment. Go slow, consider everything, and have an evaluation by a healthcare professional.

Chapter 6: Headaches That Resist Treatment and the Desperate Attempts to Crush Them

We all get headaches, but some people get a specific type that is not just painful but also life-threatening. Even babies can experience headaches, so age is not an issue.

Known as cluster headaches (CH), this specific headache can disrupt a person's daily life in almost every respect—it is one of the most debilitating headache types, and there is little treatment. Research and the search for potential treatments have led to a better understanding of this excruciatingly painful condition.

One person in every thousand suffers from cluster headache, a primary headache disorder. Each incident of a cluster headache often lasts no more than a few minutes and occurs in cycles. Aside from the usual unilateral headache, an attack may also include drooping of the eyelid, redness or discharge from the eye, and stuffiness or a runny nose on the same side as the headache.

Some refer to CHs as "suicide headaches." Since many doctors and nurses have never dealt with a CH patient, a description will assist them and everyone else in comprehending the gravity of this powerful and unbearably painful condition that many sufferers endure for the rest of their lives.

One person in one million takes their own life every year as a result of a primary headache; this number accounts for one percent of the total suicide rate. Of these, 70–80% are migraines and cluster headaches. Suicide attempts occur ten times more often than actual suicides. Compared to migraines, cluster headaches are more dangerous.

It may come as a surprise to some, but most doctors and nurses in healthcare have never dealt with a patient who has cluster headaches. Because of this, people may perceive those with cluster headaches as suffering from a mental disorder or seeking sympathy. To put it succinctly, they frequently lack credibility. Women suffer more migraine and cluster headaches than men, and, for this reason, there may be a tendency to view their symptoms as psychosomatic, requiring therapy rather than medical treatment.

Misunderstandings, drug charges, disrespect, a lack of urgency, or even a lack of education can prompt a patient to consider suicide.

Unfortunately, such incidents may occur more frequently than one might think.

Innumerable times, patients experience attacks while sitting in the emergency room for hours. Nobody on the emergency room crew has any clue how much pain they are in. Even the most basic information on this illness and its treatment is unknown to them.

Patients with CH make up only 0.1 to 0.4% of the general population. Around 7 million people worldwide and at least 400,000 in the United States suffer from this extremely rare condition.

It is well-known that cluster headache attacks cause some of the worst pain a person can feel. The extreme agony experienced by those who suffer from cluster headaches frequently makes them agitated or drowsy. Cluster headaches are characterized by intense, unilateral pain that occurs in clusters or bouts, typically centered around or behind the eyes. Tears, a stuffy or runny nose, a drooping eyelid, and facial sweating are other common symptoms that often occur on the same side as the headache. Many people report feeling a sharp or scorching pain.

Patients may notice:

Eyes are watering more than usual.

The affected eye becomes redder on the side that hurts.

The eyelids swell or droop.

Hampered vision.

Light sensitivity.

Lack of Medical Education

On average, during the four years of medical school, students spend approximately three hours learning about cluster headaches, according to physicians. The seriousness of this disorder necessitates an immediate increase in both classroom instruction and research on such medical topics. Three hours out of five thousand over the course of four years is a tiny fraction of a semester.

Ironically, medical schools in the past have also devoted little more than one hour of lecture time to diet, and yet patients are advised to discuss their diet with their primary care physician. As one healthcare professional mentioned to me, "*How am I expected to be knowledgeable about that?*"

Cluster headaches haven't received much attention in healthcare throughout their existence, but this neglect needs to change. In fact, people who suffer from these types of headaches can reach the point of suicide to obtain relief. Some patients have said, "I'd eat shoe polish if it helped relieve me of this horrible headache." Can you imagine such desperation when we live in a world of advanced healthcare, with artificial intelligence making incredible strides in diagnosis and treatment every day?

Regardless of the cause of a disorder's fatality, we must immediately increase the level of urgency to save a life. Urgency is long overdue for this group of patients. Conditions will, hopefully, gradually improve as a result of increased awareness and education.

The Search for Treatment

In desperation, patients have given up in some cases on traditional medical interventions and sought treatment outside the norm, in psychedelic drugs.

To date, some of the usual traditional treatments include:

1. Oxygen. Breathing in pure oxygen through a mask provides relief for most who use it. People feel the effects of this safe treatment within 15 minutes.

2. Triptans. When cluster headache symptoms start, doctors administer sumatriptan (Imitrex) as a shot.

3. Octreotide. Octreotide (Sandostatin), a shot of a version of the brain hormone somatostatin.

4. Local anesthetics. The numbing effect of local anesthetics, such as lidocaine, might work against cluster headache pain.

People have tried other treatments, but there is no universal agreement on a single treatment approach for all individuals. However, medicine is a specialized field that deals with individuals, and differences are inherent to it. Therefore, it would not be wise to expect one treatment for all.

Some people who suffer from this condition have found relief by using magic mushrooms. **Clusterbusters** is a patient advocacy group that claims to offer both short-term comfort and, in rare instances, long-term symptom remission. The psychoactive component in magic mushrooms, psilocybin, does not necessarily need a full-blown trip to have its effects; in fact, it is usually enough to take low amounts of the compound multiple times. The article's mention of these substances does not mean they are endorsed; it means they have helped some people.

Fifty-three individuals with cluster headaches who had sought relief through the use of psilocybin or lysergic acid diethylamide (LSD) had varied responses in terms of their symptoms. Forty-two percent of those who took psilocybin said it stopped attacks; 25 of 48 who took psilocybin and seven percent of those who took LSD said it ended cluster periods; and eighteen percent of the 19 who took psilocybin and four percent of those who took LSD said it lengthened remission periods.

This was a small sample, but hopefully, larger clinical trials with these substances will be conducted, allowing us to determine if any psychedelics are helpful in some of the patients. We cannot dismiss the utility of these drugs, as they can be beneficial for several disorders.

We must address the stigma and find acceptance for psychedelics as a new approach in medicine. Perhaps Dr. Timothy Leary of Harvard was right all along in his research, but the stigma was too ingrained for anyone to see the good in it.

Research must be thorough for these patients, as the hope is that the biology of their intractable pain and effective treatments will be discovered soon. Of course, healthcare also has a responsibility, not only in the research area but also in the **education of anyone who practices** and may encounter patients with cluster headaches. Ignorance in the area is completely unacceptable.

Chapter 7: When Is Exercise Not Exercise, and Is That Good Enough?

Working out is often thought to involve free weights, exercise programs or some other routine, but there's more to exercise than that.

Going for walks, dancing, and doing housework —although not technically exercises —every kind of movement counts toward your daily activity goal. Get more exercise to improve your health with just a straightforward adjustment.

Physical activity enhances the quality of sleep, strengthens the brain, and reduces the risk of developing certain types of cancer and heart disease. Your weekly "exercise" is the sum of all your physical activity, regardless of how long it lasts, and any movement is beneficial for your health.

According to a study published in the open access journal BMJ Open, older individuals who regularly clean up after themselves have superior memory, attention span, and leg strength. This, in turn, makes them less likely to fall.

The researchers in this study aimed to investigate whether performing home tasks among the elderly population of a developed nation would promote healthy aging and enhance cognitive and physical abilities, as this type of activity requires movement and is a measure of a person's potential to live independently.

Cooking, dusting, making the bed, ironing, hanging laundry, and washing up were all examples of light chores. Tasks such as painting and decorating, as well as heavier chores like changing the bed, vacuuming, and washing the floor, were included.

Included in the sample were 489 adults (ranging in age from 21 to 90) who were selected at random and had no cognitive impairments and fewer than five underlying medical conditions. Everyone was able to take care of their own daily needs and live independently in a residential community.

Additionally, the intensity of housework correlated with certain cognitive domains. Light housework was linked to 8% better short-term memory and 14% better long-term memory, whereas heavy housework was linked to a 14% higher attention score.

Almost two-thirds (61%, 152 younger, and 66%, 159 older) only used housework to reach the prescribed physical activity quota objective. Additionally, certain cognitive domains were linked to the level of housework intensity. After adjusting for other types of regular physical activity, the results showed a link between housework and improved physical and mental capacities. but only in the elderly population.

Researchers in Europe used a sizable database of health data from middle-aged British civil officials to conduct new investigations. Researchers monitored the employees, initially between the ages of 35 and 55, for about ten years while they completed numerous health surveys.

One of the things mentioned in the questions was doing household chores. Every task was categorized as "mild," such as cooking or doing the dishes, to "moderate" (weeding They found a link between any form of physical activity and a longer lifespan.o a longer lifespan.

What Is the Recommended Amount of Exercise?

Experts and our physicians have been telling us for years that we need to exercise, and now that we know housework can be exercise, you should feel a bit less stressed. Of course, housework may not be your total answer, but it contributes to your weekly exercise. The question remains: how much exercise should you be getting and whether you should do intense things or be a bit more casual about them?

Intensity has benefits for some, especially regarding the activity, but you should keep in mind that any exercise is good. As long as you're not spending the entire day sitting in a chair, watching television, playing a board game, or doing something else, you can count your exercise credits. Guidelines are available online for those of us who need a bit more help establishing the correct amount for ourselves.

Keep something else in mind, too. When you perceive an activity as more than a task or obligation, it can significantly impact your motivation. When we consider exercise to be a chore like housework, it becomes something you feel obligated to do. However, when you consider both housework and exercise as beneficial for your mental health, cognitive abilities, and longevity, they become valuable investments.

Always remind yourself that you are doing this for yourself, even if required. The benefits are threefold: required work, exercise, and longevity. When did you ever think of housework as providing additional years of life for you? Not only does housework involve exercise and longevity, but it also combats anxiety and depression, thereby enhancing our mood.

You probably hated housework, but a new light is shining on it, and you should let it shine.

Chapter 8: Psychotherapy That Is Pseudoscience According to Professionals: Conversion Therapy

Not all "therapies" that are offered are bona fide psychotherapies, according to experts and the American Psychiatric Association.

Psychotherapy has proven to be beneficial to many who seek help with everyday issues or a mental health diagnosis, but not all "therapies" are legitimate and based on solid research. When we begin to examine some of them, they don't hold up because they are based on myths, unproven theories, or outright nonsense. One of the prime examples of pseudoscientific "therapies" for LGBTQ individuals is conversion therapy.

Allegedly intended to "cure" homosexuality, the methods and the history of this "therapy" are shocking and criminal in their entirety. The soothsayers backing these "cures" went to extreme measures in a frantic effort to bring these gay individuals back into the fold as it were. For example, "Eugen Steinach, a pioneering Austrian endocrinologist, believed homosexuality was rooted in a man's testicles. This theory led to testicle transplantation experiments in the 1920s during which gay men were castrated and then given "heterosexual" testicles".

Freud took a less drastic approach and believed homosexuality was related to a problem in arrested sexual development and that it was a matter of conditioning that needed to be addressed. Therefore, it is not a "disease" but an inappropriate resolution of unconscious conflicts.

Zealots, on missions to cleanse the world of sin, came up with their theories and saw it as everything from devil possession to a failure in faith to serious mental illness. The world of science played a backseat role in most of this and dismissed it as a mental disorder until professionals determined it was not a mental disorder, disease, or crime. The history of this journey to a change in mental health orientation is lengthy, but extensive books and articles are now available.

Anyone deemed homosexual was subjected to horrific "medical" procedures by some who used electric shock to the brain or sex organs, lobotomies, exposure to heterosexual pornography, and myriad brutal or unthinkable "therapies" to bring the person back to what they perceived as "normal" sexual functioning.

It wasn't until Evelyn Hooker, in 1953, working at the National Institute of Mental Health, began research on "normal homosexuals" that resulted in much-needed change. In 1973, the American Psychiatric Association removed homosexuality as a disorder from DSM-III. The book is considered the essential psychiatry manual for diagnosing mental illnesses, and if one has been removed, it is for good reason.

Organizations devoted to maintaining the law and human rights have become involved in disclosing the true nature of conversion therapy, also known as reparative or sexual reorientation therapy. One, the SPLC has indicated, "This practice — which can include violent role play, reenactment of past abuses, and exercises involving nudity and intimate touching — has been discredited by virtually all major American medical, psychiatric, psychological, and professional counseling organizations."

Despite the vigorous response of professional healthcare organizations against it, the practice remains in use today at private clinics and practices where homosexuality is treated and explained as it was over one hundred years ago. Not only is this unethical, it may be criminal and could expose these individuals to charges against them. However, it presents itself as a way to "cure" the individual and potentially save their souls. If insurance is involved, questions may arise about the diagnosis given for "treatment." If government funds are used, there is another consideration and involvement for investigation.

One thing that everyone must keep in mind is that not everyone who offers mental health services has a license from a state licensing agency. There are those who present themselves as mental health professionals who are neither educated nor licensed for the task. Any consideration of therapy necessitates personal research; wall plaques, impressive letterheads, or affiliations with any group are not sufficient.

A patient's family once told a colleague that their adult son was flashing young girls at a local school, and they wanted treatment for him. He had already been arrested once. He was referred to a psychiatrist, who said that for $10,000 he could guarantee a "cure." Guess what happened when the young man continued to offend? The psychiatrist admitted he had no experience with the disorder.

I have worked in large psychiatric hospitals where staff who were providing group therapy believed in demonic possession. One staff member told someone with a diagnosis of schizophrenia that he wasn't praying or fasting enough. The management also allowed purported religious chaplains to visit our units and provide treatment advice, despite their lack of qualifications. One woman, who wore clerical garb, was a former patient at another facility and not "clergy" at all, but she fooled the staff.

At another major hospital in the Midwest, they don't require licensing for professionals who engage in questionable "therapy." I know of another hospital where a religious group came in to "visit" patients who were taken, singularly, into a visiting room where exorcisms were performed until a vigilant staff member discovered it and refused entrance to the group again.

One unscrupulous analytic school sent their students to psychiatric hospitals, where they presented themselves as "friendly visitors" to patients whom they were "treating" analytically. The administrator responsible for visitor privileges knew nothing about this practice, but a psychologist uncovered it, and the school was told this was no longer permitted. How many of these "visitors" are still going to hospitals and presenting themselves as friends or religious group members offering solace to the lonely patients?

Conversion therapy is still being offered, and it is still considered pseudoscience and is not recognized as any type of treatment by mental health professionals. Homosexuality is not a disorder, a moral failure, or a changeable choice. Anyone in the LGBTQ community needs to know that they are not "sick" or immoral. Therapy is for personal issues or social stigma, not "conversion."

Chapter 9:
Rapunzel Wasn't Simply in a Castle; It's a Psychiatric Syndrome

Remember the maiden told to *"let down your hair"* so the prince could climb to reach her? Yup, there's more to that.

The girl with the long hair from the Grimm Brothers' 1812 fairy tale inspired the name for a syndrome. Because the fairy tale and the clinical cases documented in a 1968 paper shared traits—the patient's unusually long hair and the rarity of the occurrence—the condition was dubbed Rapunzel syndrome. Medical professionals didn't describe the disorder until 1889, despite documenting the first trichobezoar case in 1779.

For ages, people have recognized undigested masses in the stomachs of animals and humans as bezoars (accumulations of foreign material in the stomach). However, this discovery has increased in frequency. Despite the prevalence of information, Rapunzel syndrome is still quite rare and considered a form of obsessive-compulsive disorder (OCD).

Researchers have recorded 24 cases in the literature, with a mean age of 10.8 years. Among these cases, there is one male patient and 23 female patients. Patients often report symptoms such as nausea, vomiting, and discomfort in the abdomen, as well as indicators of blockage.

The disorder is not only a medical concern but can cause death in extreme situations, such as in young girls who have eaten excessive amounts of their hair. Trichotillomania involves hair pulling, which is not fatal but can cause bald spots. It is not unusual for surgical removal of the hairballs to be necessary because this hair may cause intestinal blockages.

As a symptom of trichotillomania, an individual may bite their nails, chew their lips, or pick at their skin, scalp, eyebrows, or other areas of their body. Though tweezers or other implements can be used, people typically remove hair by hand.

Some people have rituals around selecting hair and pulling it; for instance, after combing one's hands through the hair, the individual may look for coarse hair toward the front of the hairline. Some people, after having their hair plucked, may examine it closely and then eat some of it.

Hair loss in household items, such as clothing or blankets, as well as in dogs or dolls, can indicate something more severe in terms of psychopathology. Because hair is a non-nutritive substance, we might also think of this as a form of pica.

Engaging in hair-pulling in private is common, and an episode can last from a few seconds to hours. Usually, individuals with this disorder attempt to hide it from others, but the signs may become evident once the balding patches, skin scabs, and chewed-down nails are obvious.

Causes of the Disorder

Trichotillomania typically begins in adolescence, between the ages of 10 and 13, and continues far into late adolescence, but it can last a lifetime. Most times, babies' hair loss is minimal and resolves without medical intervention.

Genetics may influence the development of trichotillomania. Having a close family member who suffers from the disorder might increase the risk of developing it.

Some people have trichotillomania as a reaction to extremely stressful events or situations; others find that boredom, solitude, and privacy make them more likely to pull their hair out. The exact cause, however, is not clear.

The complex nature of trichotillomania necessitates a multi-pronged approach to prevention, diagnosis, and therapy. Primary care physicians, dermatologists, psychiatrists, and licensed clinical psychologists may see the patient. Therapy methods and possibly medication will be part of the treatment plan. Treatments for trichotillomania that are presently under research include habit reversal training and cognitive-behavioral therapy (CBT).

Although the disorder primarily affects adolescent females, adults may also engage in this behavior in stressful situations. I have observed adult female healthcare professionals playing with their hair. Although I did not see any active hair pulling, there was hair twisting and manipulation that was not intended for styling purposes. This may make it clearer that the behavior is not constant but may be episodic and persist into adulthood, where behavior modification may be effective.

Chapter 10: Kindness and Charity Benefit Us More Than We Know

The secret is out, and it's that we are the gainers, too, when we give and promote kindness to others.

Kindness and special consideration for others who may be in need physically or mentally shouldn't be limited to certain times of the year. Goodness is something all of us should be exhibiting all year round, and we all benefit from it.

Do we need research to tell us that we will receive something wonderful in return for thinking of others in their time of need? If that's what anyone needs to help them rethink their behavior, OK, bring it on.

Literature and films all laud the heartwarming aspects of charity and caring for our brothers and sisters worldwide, regardless of religious beliefs. Watching a classic like "It's a Wonderful Life" renews our belief in the potential for positive change. How many saw Mary Bailey as the true hero here and failed to give her the due she deserved? Well, a WAPO columnist did.

Many of us will watch the several iterations of the film "A Christmas Carol" and see what pushes Scrooge to repent his miserly actions and channel the true spirit of Christmas. But first, the three ghosts of Christmas must terrorize Scrooge. Who knew it had ghosts, or are they simply spirits? I'll leave that to the literature scholars.

The season is a time of sharing, goodwill, and charity. Whether it's a religious holiday (or holy day) isn't the issue here. Human dignity and fair treatment of others are the emphases.

Those who celebrate Kwanzaa have returned to the true essence of the season, where the cost of a gift isn't the issue (really, a Lexus?), and it should be replaced with a gift made for the receiver.

I've worked in mental health centers where patients, who had been in psychiatric hospitals for decades, didn't know what an appropriate Christmas gift might be. One man gave someone a pound of raw bacon, and he was a bit unnerved that he didn't receive a hearty thanks for it. Another patient gave a single Bic pen wrapped in Christmas paper to a worker. The joy exhibited was moving.

The writer O'Henry enriched our reading and the spirit of love in difficult times when he wrote "The Gift of the Magi." If you haven't read it, you have a link here. Of course, in my readings, someone asked why one of the kings brought the gift of myrrh, an oil that is used for the solemn procedures before burial. Again, the scholars can debate.

Enter the Research

Research hasn't failed us in providing proof that giving is as beneficial to the recipient as the giver and perhaps more so. One form of charity doesn't have the effect we would expect, and it's anxiety.

The so-called checkout charity solicitations often bring anxiety, and their "results caution managers that checkout charity solicitations may have unintended consequences on customers that result in negative encounter outcomes, particularly in service environments in which the solicitation is technology-mediated." Supermarkets often ask me to "round up" my order for charity. Pharmacy chains do this as well.

Guess what one incredible benefit of giving can be. You might be interested in a study indicating that charitable giving can promote a longer life. That's like paying it forward big time.

This study indicates that "older people who are helpful to others reduce their risk of dying by nearly 60 percent compared to peers who provide neither practical help nor emotional support to relatives, help neighbors or friends." Maybe we should have plaques with "*Give Unto Others and Prolong Your Life.*"

Altruism does affect us by lowering our stress hormone levels and thereby increasing our immune system's ability to protect us. Good? Charitable works have the potential to tame cancer, making it a more beneficial endeavor. Volunteering is a wonderful way to help others, so money is not the issue.

All of us need a sense of worth and belonging to our culture. Research out of an Alzheimer's center indicated that volunteering and giving of ourselves may help stave off neurological illness, heart disease, and stroke. Once again, the reward for the giver comes in the form of improved health indicators.

When we feel our lives and activities have been limited, there is time for charitable works either via the internet or some other activity. Think about it.

Chapter 11: Cancer or Cognition: Where Does Nicotine Lie and Why the Controversy?

Cherry-picking research specifics has always been the bane of researchers, authors, and corporations, and when we consider nicotine, the same nexus of controversy exists. How can we resolve this issue and distinguish the important information from the irrelevant? That is the task all of us must engage in to be sure we're choosing wisely.

When corporations begin expounding on the positive side of nicotine and fail to mention, equally, the dangers, we must be ever vigilant. This, of course, applies, especially when younger individuals are the target audience for these products. Want an example? Think of vaping, which is not without its dangers of inhaling dangerous materials directly into the lungs.

Of course, we know that nicotine has a role in cognition, but is it such a significant role that to deny someone nicotine's benefits would be unacceptable? Is nicotine vital for cognition? Doubtless, it does have a role within specific biologically determined guidelines set by our bodies' needs.

Nicotine is a natural product found in our bodies, and, in fact, we do have receptors that naturally respond to it. Therefore, it is not alien to us, but when we introduce excess nicotine, what happens? And the mode of introduction may have an impact on our health.

Much of the research, in the past, has concentrated on cigarette smoking and nicotine's effect, or the impact on lung and stomach cancers. However, our progress has been significant, albeit not sufficient. New products are producing nicotine in ways that can be both addictive and dangerous to health, but they are emphasizing cognitive benefits. I find this disingenuous and an apt example of cherry-picking.

Anti-smoking campaigns have been directed at adults and, more recently, at younger smokers. But cigarettes are not the only products, as I've mentioned, that deliver nicotine directly into the body via the lungs and stomach. We have had nicotine pouches for years, and, unfortunately, some prominent sports figures have been known to use these.

Placing the pouch between the cheek and jaw releases nicotine and, in some cases, a sweetener as a stimulant. Still, it also has another horrifying effect—jaw cancer, which can result in head and neck cancer and death. We must ask ourselves how any such product could be used within safe limits.

However, the effects of nicotine extend beyond the head and neck, as major cancer centers across the United States have reported its impact on brain development, cardiovascular issues, and oral health.

In accordance with the requirements of the Family Smoking Prevention and Tobacco Control Act of 2009, the Food and Drug Administration (FDA) confirmed that at least one marketed item fulfilled the public health standard. Under this criterion, the products' potential advantages and harms to the general public are taken into account. Shouldn't such items be considered a recreational product rather than one that is needed? If that's the case, motivation is the issue, and advertising and promotion will push these products to an eagerly anticipating younger public.

The evaluation by the agency found that the authorized products have a lower risk of cancer and other serious health conditions compared to cigarettes and most smokeless tobacco products, including moist snuff, because they contain substantially fewer harmful constituents. Note the word "fewer." Furthermore, the applicant presented research that demonstrated a significant percentage of adult smokers and users of smokeless tobacco products made the transition to the newly allowed nicotine pouch products.

Please note that whenever we are using materials for researching consumer opinions, the subjectivity is shaky in terms of validity regarding what is being researched. And, what's more, the questions are also open to reasonable concern. Phrasing and positioning questions are everything.

The reasoning here does not present a solid belief that these products are totally safe. Note that the products were indicated to have a lower risk of cancer and other serious health conditions. The statement did not suggest the absence of cancer risk, but rather its reduction. Therefore, we can assume that cancer is still one of the resulting health concerns from using these products.

Making the Case for Nicotine

There is no question that nicotine does have a notable effect on the brain and, possibly, not only working memory but also attention span. Such properties would make it highly attractive, especially to students.

Studies with cigarette smoking are primarily where we receive this information. Smoking may affect levels of brain-derived neurotrophic factor (BDNF), according to these studies. To this day, we still do not know how nicotine modifies brain chemistry and how it specifically impacts BDNF and cognition.

One of the studies revealed an interesting result: extended nicotine abstinence negatively impacted cognitive performance as BDNF levels declined. If we consider this information crucial, it would suggest that the promotion of continued use of nicotine products is advantageous. Withdrawing from the product has detrimental effects on mood and memory, just like with any addiction.

Overall, we must consider the potential dangers of anything that we use — hair dyes, food, colorings, medications, and recreational products such as nicotine-based materials. But when it comes to influencing younger users, we have a moral obligation to them to provide guidance, information, and involvement in any FDA approvals.

Chapter 12: Medical Devices Are Under Cyberattacks, and Your Life Could Be at Risk

The prevalence of ransomware attacks against hospitals and potentially patient medical devices has made cybersecurity a pressing issue.

The hearts of millions of patients worldwide beat and are monitored by implanted medical devices that can be programmed externally, and therein lies the potential threat to their lives. And it's more extensive and not limited to these devices.

The number of pacemakers in the world was about 1.14 million in 2016. By 2023, that figure was projected to rise to 1.43 million. While it affords life-giving relief to these patients, it also places them at risk because of a healthcare failure to anticipate how to protect patients from cyberattacks.

Every piece of equipment, from hospital beds to infusion pumps to monitors that measure and track vital signs, is connected, and since everything is online, it is all theoretically hackable. Too many devices utilize commercial software that is readily susceptible to viruses and worms.

Until recently, manufacturers were not required to provide patches or other solutions to their customers when vulnerabilities on older devices surfaced. The current troublesome situations may not be receiving enough attention, as evidenced by the fact that these attacks are not limited to healthcare. Recently, cyberattacks have also targeted museums.

A ransomware attack against Museum Software Solutions provider Gallery Systems, which includes the Museum of Modern Art in New York, the Crystal Bridges Museum of Modern Art, the Metropolitan Museum of Art, and the Chrysler Museum of Art, among others, has caused operational disruptions at online museums.

Hospital ransomware attacks are proving to be a serious threat to their operations, patient records, and healthcare in general. In 2023, statistics indicate that attacks targeted about 141 hospitals. One massive data breach compromised the records of 11 million patients at HCA Healthcare and should serve as a stark reminder of how the nation's largest healthcare organizations' defenses can be breached.

One of the largest non-profit health systems in the United States, Common Spirit Healthcare, disclosed that their breach compromised over 600,000 records. The attack caused disruptions to some hospitals' operations and cost approximately $160 million in losses.

Congress asserted that the body most responsible for monitoring and providing solutions to this imminent danger was the FDA. In September 2023, the FDA published final guidance on pre-market submissions; however, the advice is focused on newly authorized medical devices and lacks provisions for protecting older products already on the market.

What happens to all those unprotected patients with older implants? Should we bring them to the OR for a device upgrade? What is the general policy regarding hospital data protection? We advise anyone with questions to contact the FDA at ocod@fda.hhs.gov for further information.

Could prescription-assistant programs or glucose-monitoring devices also be vulnerable to dangers not anticipated at this point? Anything that goes over an open network or Bluetooth can be a target.

Currently, every hospital administrator in the nation must be asking themselves which massive computer program they are using for all their data and whether it is sufficiently encrypted or protected in some way. How many healthcare programs engage with non-protected entities in the medical field? Identify the biggest player in healthcare. Investigate and gain knowledge.

The situation is dire, and solutions can't wait for some computer guru to write a new encryption program. How many think tanks are lasering in on the issues of life and death in healthcare, and how far along are they in implementing their resolutions?

Chapter 13: Doing Nothing, Including No 10K Steps, Is Good for Mental Health

Too often, we adhere to mandated wellness tips, some of which are baseless, to help maintain our mental and creative abilities. Forget much of it.

It's natural to feel overburdened and constantly on the go in today's demanding world. We frequently place more importance on getting things done, multitasking, and being active than on pausing to unwind, which may be regulated by the default mode network. But according to research, doing nothing — even something as straightforward as taking a break or a leisurely walk — can be really beneficial for our mental health.

While we're at it, let's put the idea of needing to take 10,000 steps a day to maintain our health to rest. Where did it come from, and is it true? No, there apparently is no scientific evidence to support this idea, which "appears to have started as a marketing strategy by a Japanese pedometer company in the 1960s." Got it? Do you feel more at ease about not reaching those 10K steps every day?

Now, let's talk about rights. We forget the right to do nothing, including the 10K steps. The United Nations has a Universal Declaration of Human Rights that indicates that *"Everyone has the right to rest and leisure, including reasonable limitations of working hours and periodic holidays with pay."* If the UN thinks such restrictions should apply worldwide, why wouldn't we toss aside our guilt about rest and leisure (aka doing nothing at all)? If I said it was in your best interest for optimal health, would it be easier to do?

The act of "doing nothing," or things that require little mental effort, gives our brains a chance to rest and refuel. It permits us to become relaxed and let our brains roam, or what some call daydreaming, whether creative or not. What do we receive when we allow ourselves to do nothing and think for pleasure? Reduced stress levels and a general sense of peace can result from this.

But one study says the issue is that people undervalue sitting and thinking, which makes them feel they must be doing something. *"These results suggest an inherent difficulty in accurately appreciating how engaging just thinking can be and could explain why people prefer keeping themselves busy rather than taking a moment for reflection and imagination in our daily lives."*

Taking a leisurely stroll is a well-known activity that is frequently linked to mental health. Walking has many physical advantages, such as bettering cardiovascular health and enhancing stamina, but it also offers advantages for our mental health and even creativity.

We may unplug from our devices and the relentless demands of our everyday lives by going for a stroll. It offers us an opportunity to re-engage with nature, pay attention to our surroundings, and unwind. Walking can be contemplative because of its repetitive motion, which encourages mindfulness and lowers anxiety. It even has an effect on our weight-promoting genes.

Our creativity can grow when we do nothing. We give our minds room to expand with new thoughts and viewpoints when we allow ourselves to take a break from continual stimulation and distractions. Throughout history, many great thinkers and creators have emphasized the significance of solitude and downtime as sources of inspiration.

It's crucial to understand that being inactive does not imply being ineffective or lazy. It involves purposefully blocking off time to rejuvenate. While active hobbies and regular exercise have their benefits, it's just as important to schedule time for stillness and relaxation.

Our mental health can be greatly improved by accepting the idea of doing nothing, even if it just involves taking a break or taking a leisurely walk. It boosts creativity, eases stress, and improves general well-being by allowing our minds to rest. A happier and more balanced way of living can result from incorporating these quiet periods into our regular lives.

Chapter 14: Exercise in Outdoor Greenery Has an Important Effect on MH and Brain

Is there a difference between exercising outdoors or indoors in virtual greenery related to mental and physical health?

A study from the United Nations says that by 2050, 68% of the world's people may live in cities. Only 33% of people lived in cities around the world in 1950, so the increase is a vast and quick rise in a short amount of time. This level of urbanization has quickly changed the environment from an evolutionary point of view. For example, people who live in cities see fewer wild areas, more traffic, and more pollution in the air and water. This lack of access to wild areas, a.k.a. "green areas," can have wonderful effects on our brain, mental health, and physiology.

Corporations have been leading us to believe that exercise indoors is a great way to engage in these activities, whether through an inability to access the outdoors or an inclination to remain inside. Researchers, however, have not found that exercising indoors provides all the benefits associated with exercising outdoors.

The research is quite specific in how outdoor activities activate portions of our brain involved in maintaining tranquility and engaging in problem-solving activities. Many of us have seen the 10-second commercials with calming outdoor sounds. The sounds of nature have a primal reaction that we should use to our benefit.

Being outside has been an important part of human development for thousands of years. Because of this, it is possible that the ways people react to nature will stay the same. There is not much evidence that the structure of the human brain has changed in the last 4,000 years. But it has been challenging for scientists to agree on how these effects happen until now. The research over the last few decades indicates the benefits of these sounds.

One study looked into how looking at forest scenery affects the amount of oxygenated hemoglobin in the brain. The green atmosphere was different from the scenery of cities. The authors saw a big drop in oxygenated hemoglobin in one brain area when people looked at pictures of forests. To help with problem-solving, this area tends to become more active when you are doing mentally demanding chores.

Few studies have looked at how forest therapy changes brain function. In a study and others that have been done before, changes in brain activity while being in a forest were measured by looking at the concentration of hemoglobin in the part of the brain that handles higher processes, like decision-making and problem-solving.

The researchers found that looking at real forests relaxes the body by reducing oxygen in the right part of the brain. Research of this type would support the premise that exercising indoors and viewing a monitor that shows outdoor forest areas is an effective means to provide what the brain perceives as "natural" and, therefore, useful to help us relieve stress and attain relaxation.

A short walk through a forest or just taking a moment to enjoy the view has been linked to lower cortisol levels and heart rate. Green space has been linked to better sleep, lower blood pressure, and a lower chance of chronic diseases. This advantage is probably because people who spend more time in green spaces also say they exercise more.

What are the consequences of depriving adults or children of access to real forest environments? We now know that something called nature-deficit disorder, linked to living in cities, has grown into a major social issue. People with this disorder spend less time outside than people did in the past.

Interesting ways to address this disorder, especially with children, include

Have a meal outside with your friends. Bring a blanket or towel, and eat lunch outside.

Watch the clouds. Look up to see how fast they are moving. Ask the kids to describe the shapes they see in the clouds. What do the different types of clouds mean in terms of our weather? Ask children to identify them.

Watch the birds. Ask kids to count the variety of animals they can spot. The "Seek" app by "iNaturalist" (https://www.inaturalist.org/pages/seek_app) can help you figure out what kind of animal or plant you are looking at.

Put out a bird feeder and watch the different kinds of birds that come to it. For people who are allergic to nuts, the process can be as easy as getting some pine cones and spreading peanut butter or shortening on them. Add some birdseed on top. Help them hang it from a tree branch or just put it outside a window.

I had bird feeders installed at a nursing home where residents lay in bed all day, staring out the window. The residents began to discuss the birds they had seen and the activities they were watching, which was amazing. It was a decision to change the way they spent their days.

Get some flowers or a tree and plant them together. It does not matter how big or small your job is. Save an avocado pit and grow it into a tree in your home. You can plant it in your yard. Planting is a wonderful way to learn about and take care of nature.

Go on treasure hunts in nature. Find nature where you are. Record what you find using your phone or a cheap camera. Some examples of searches and activities include:

Gather leaves. Ask kids to count how many different kinds of leaves they can find. Help them make rubbings of leaves to showcase their outdoor activities as art.

Get a light-colored sheet or towel and put it down next to a bush on the ground. Shake the sheet to see what falls from the bush onto it. (A hand lens would be very helpful here.)

Go on a "Square Foot Adventure." Find a small area of grass or dirt that is about 1 square foot and mark it. Lay down and take a good look. What lives there?

Students should write about nature. Tell kids to draw something intriguing about nature and add a few words or lines to describe it. Tell the kids to add to this tableau every time they go outside.

Find art in the outdoors. Take a picture adventure together. To get young people to take shots of interesting rocks, flowers, grasses, insects, and other things in nature.

Play games outside with each other. Catch the Flag, Tag, Red Light, Green Light, Mother May I.

Play Nature Bingo together. You can find a large number of Nature Bingo cards online or create your own.

Researchers have found that people with a better connection to nature are less stressed and anxious and visit public green spaces more often. Clarifying the link between these two factors is crucial for individuals with a weaker connection to nature. Researchers could explore this intriguing connection, which raises questions about our psychological bond with nature. Daydreaming about being in a forest might also serve our need for immersion in a natural environment.

Would it work? Let's see what the researchers think about that one. Of course, this could be an activity we engage in while meditating, and it may contribute to the existing literature on the benefits of meditation.

The green space is waiting for you; what are you waiting for?

Chapter 15: Are You Writing in Cursive or On a Computer? It may make a difference in your creativity. What do/did the "greats" use?

An exquisitely sharpened point on a Blackwing 602 pencil slides smoothly across the paper. Laying down a carefully constructed sentence and then paragraphs and pages, it is the beginning work of a premier writer. The writer, of course, was Truman Capote, who admitted that he was "... a completely horizontal author."

Each draft of his writings followed a set pattern, first composed in cursive on yellow paper rather than on a typewriter. He jotted down his thoughts and then revised them in penciled cursive. A second go-round was also with the preferred writing implement, the Blackwing, whose lead gave life to his verse.

The third draft, again on yellow paper, would not be written by hand. "No, I don't get out of bed to do this. I balance the machine on my knees. Sure, it works fine; I can manage a hundred words in a minute. Well, when the yellow draft is finished, I put the manuscript away for a while, a week, a month, sometimes longer... If all goes well, I type the final version on white paper, and that's that."

Literary historians, who have cataloged the path Capote took, noted all of the turns in the journey. However, his use of cursive writing receives neither a mention nor a thoughtful moment given to his use of cursive writing.

Capote's cursive was never considered as instrumental in his creativity and was dismissed as something authors use. The East Indian proverb comes to mind: "The eye does not see what the mind does not know."

Some of Capote's most famous and fretted-about work (Answered Prayers) never did reach his publisher's office. Advance after advance would not budge the man who had lost his creative fire in a sea of addiction. He left the Blackwings behind.

Atwood and Other Writers

Margaret Atwood, best known for her "The Handmaid's Tale," is a prolific writer of novels, poems, and essays. Her creative process also includes using Le Crayon.

"*My absolute opening entry is always a handheld object with a point on one end. So it's going to be either a pencil or a pen. And then it is applied to a flat substance of some kind, which is usually a piece of paper but could be a piece of cardboard if one's stuck without the paper. Or even my arm when things get really bad.*"

Atwood, of course, loves a sense of humor, and she has indicated that when a pen or pencil isn't available, she conjures up visions of using other things. "*... having that moment and finding that you're unable to set it down except with a knife on your leg or something. You actually don't want to do that. So I recommend the paper and pencil. Or if you must, some other stylus writing device that provides a permanent record of what you just set down.*" But a pencil or pen would be preferable.

Vladimir Nabokov, like Capote, also preferred using the Blackwing 602 from Eberhardt Faber for outlining his novels on index cards.

Hemingway never stated a preference but had a particular perspective on pencils. "*Writing at first in pencil gives you one-third more chance to improve it. That is .333, which is a damn good average for a hitter.*" It also maintains fluidity for a longer duration, allowing you to perform better and with greater ease.

The sentence may be somewhat awkward, but it conveys the idea that a pencil offers three distinct perspectives on writing. Hemingway had other advice for the new writer in his A Movable Feast when he said, "*...the blue-backed notebooks, the two pencils and the pencil sharpener (a public pocketknife was too wasteful), the marble-topped tables, the smell of café crammed, the smell of early-morning sweeping out and mopping, and luck were all you needed.*"

People say that John Steinbeck always started his writing sessions with 24 Blackwing pencils. However, he also used the Mongol 480 and was said to have used 300 pencils to write one of his best-known tomes, East of Eden and 60 for The Grapes of Wrath and Cannery Row.

Did Steinbeck write with all of those pencils or break them in frustration or a flurry of creativity? No one will ever know.

Judy Blume feels that she produces her best work when she has a pencil in hand. Her thoughts on the process? "*Whatever it is that happens between the brain and the pencil in my hand, that's really important to my process.*"

Pen enthusiasts include Neil Gaiman, Simone de Beauvoir, Stephen King, Dylan Thomas, Jane Austen (who used a quill pen and iron gall ink), Charles Dickens, J. K. Rowling, Arthur Conan Doyle, Sylvia Plath, and Claire Messud.

Little is known of all the famous writers who used either pencils or pens of various types, but the implement used in the process was uniquely involved. Now we know what it is.

Why Cursive? What Does It Do?

I find cursive with a pencil, with the lead that isn't hard, to be a sensual experience. There's something about that smooth traverse across the paper in precise cursive that brings a feeling of contentment and pleasure. In that, I believe I'm not alone. Did I know my creativity and cursive went hand-in-hand with portions of my brain? No, I didn't.

Researchers have been interested in whether or not using technology such as computer laptops vs. longhand note writing might have some effect on learning and memory since it might affect different areas of the brain. Several studies have looked at this process and indicate that laptops may impair learning because of distraction. But what does that say about creativity?

Creativity is involved in language and the richness of language, which is available to the writer. Language development areas of the brain are directly affected by cursive writing, as has been shown by research

Cursive handwriting is a brain trainer or a gym for creativity, insight, working memory, and language production. It may improve your ability to bring multiple areas of the brain into play, adding to your cognitive abilities.

Research has shown that first graders who learned to write in cursive received higher scores in reading words and in spelling than a comparable group.

"One possible explanation is the continuity of movement in cursive, whereas, in manuscript writing, attention is given to single letters. The continuous line in writing a word provides kinesthetic feedback about the shape of the words as a whole, which is absent in manuscript writing."

The benefits of cursive go further in that it promotes left-brain thinking, language, and memory. Evidence indicates that it also improves problem-solving abilities and helps to integrate visual and tactile information as well as fine-motor skills.

Are you ready to begin writing your outlines, short stories, and poems in cursive again? The research is convincing, and who among us wouldn't want a bit more firepower in our writing arsenal? I would.

Chapter 16: The Mind and Body May Respond to Acupuncture, Which Appears to Be Effective

Many areas of medicine are using acupuncture, and it even shows promise in treating PTSD. The world of medicine is also showing more interest in it as a treatment modality.

The ancient art of acupuncture, which is theorized to work by potentially inhibiting certain nerve pathways, may be a means of releasing bodily tensions. It is now being investigated as a treatment for PTSD.

What is acupuncture, and how is it used in medicine? Acupuncture involves inserting thin, solid metal needles into the skin. The acupuncturist's hands move in a specific way or use electricity to stimulate the needles. The more modern belief regarding acupuncture is that it can stimulate portions of the central nervous system and, therefore, produce results in specific instances. The results are believed to be caused by enabling the body's own health-protective aspects to begin initiating action to regain health.

Traditional Chinese medicine uses acupuncture as a form of healthcare. Practitioners think the body has more than 2,000 acupuncture points linked together by meridians. Energy, known as Qi (pronounced "chee"), flows through the body via these pathways. Qi is what generally keeps the body healthy. Body disorders result from problems with the flow of energy, which can then cause diseases.

Studies have looked into how effective acupuncture can be for treating neck and shoulder pain, facial pain, fibromyalgia pain, and helping post-stroke patients improve their communication.

However, many of the meta-analysis studies that have been performed appear to be primarily professional articles in Chinese journals. This doesn't mean acupuncture can't help Western medicine, but it may only show how much it's used in alternative medicine. By looking at evidence maps and summaries of SRs (systematic reviews of therapies) on acupuncture, beneficial therapies appear to exist. And the therapy has been adopted by many nations worldwide.

A 2013 WHO report indicates that 103 of its member countries have allowed the use of acupuncture. A World Federation of Acupuncture-Moxibustion Societies survey found that 183 (91%) of the 202 countries they looked at used acupuncture. Additionally, 178 (93%) of the 192 UN member countries have acupuncture practices, and 59 (31%) have insurance coverage for some or all of acupuncture.

People often seek relief from pain. About 43% of adults in the UK, or 28 million people, have chronic pain, and for 7.9 million of those adults, the pain is moderately or seriously limiting. About 62% of people over 75 have chronic pain, which is higher than the rate in younger age groups.

People who are in pain often have a very low quality of life because it makes it challenging for them to work, socialize, sleep, and keep up relationships. It can also make them depressed, less motivated, and less active. Because of this, constant pain is a major problem for healthcare services and government policy. And pain is a concern for major corporations.

One area of research that is receiving more interest is migraine. Individuals suffering from migraines frequently experience moderate-to-severe throbbing headaches, accompanied by phobic reactions to light and sound, nausea, and vomiting. During acute attacks, migraines can make it difficult for people to go about their daily lives and do their jobs.

In this study, compared to sham acupuncture, real acupuncture sometimes produced relief in ten minutes, reduced the number of migraine days, lowered the amount of medicine needed, and improved quality of life. The relief from acupuncture lasted for up to three months, but it appears to have been ineffective a year after the treatment ended.

More and more people are interested in acupuncture as a safe and successful treatment that does not involve drugs. Several studies on migraine have indicated that acupuncture is a better way to treat it than fake acupuncture and regular treatment. It also greatly lowers the number of migraines that happen and starts working faster than oral medication.

A randomized clinical study with people who had advanced cancer found that both acupuncture and massage helped with pain relief, fatigue, insomnia, and quality of life over 26 weeks. There was no significant difference between the two treatments, though.

According to research, problems like back or neck pain, knee pain from osteoarthritis, and pain after surgery may all benefit from acupuncture. Additionally, it might help ease the pain in the joints that comes from taking aromatase inhibitors, which are medicines that people with breast cancer take.

A review of data from 20 studies involving 6,376 people with painful conditions such as back pain, osteoarthritis, neck pain, or headaches showed that acupuncture continued to help with all but neck pain for a year after the final treatment ended. Other areas where acupuncture may be helpful are seasonal allergy complaints, stress incontinence in women, and cancer patients' nausea and vomiting. Despite its potential to alleviate asthma symptoms, acupuncture has not demonstrated any improvement in lung function.

Overall, there is a wealth of research worldwide to indicate that acupuncture has a place in traditional medicine, provided that it is utilized by a well-qualified healthcare professional. The variety of disorders and illnesses that may benefit from acupuncture is increasing with more research in various areas of health. The hope is, therefore, that it may prove more beneficial and even surpass some forms of pharmacologic intervention. However, there is yet to be proof of the latter.

Chapter 17: Skinnier, Sicker? Weight-Loss Meds' Raise Concerns

These drugs don't advertise or emphasize their physical side effects, but people are starting to notice them.

Taking any type of medicine always carries a risk, with some risks being more concerning than others. If you look at the Physicians' Desk Reference (available online) and navigate to the side effects section, you may be surprised by the lengthy lists of side effects for some medications. However, when examining the area of specific concern, the "rare" effects, it is essential to consider how few people will likely experience them. It's probably not many, but you must be wary if you're one of them.

Many of us may take multiple medications daily, and we depend on our prescriber's ability to monitor those that are safe for us and exclude those that may be problematic. Anyone who wishes to be safer may do a bit of their research, and that's fine. It does not mean you are suspicious; you only wish to ensure there's no problem.

There are hundreds of medications on the list, and it's nearly impossible for anyone to know if one of those uncommon side effects could affect you. It is, therefore, in your best interest to be vigilant for these effects. In addition to being aware of the side effects, most patients would not know that the number of side effects may increase as the number of people taking the medication increases. Not every side effect manifests immediately, and it may require a significant increase in medication usage for it to show up.

How does a side effect enter the PDR? Usually, during clinical trials where drugs are being tested on patients, the principal investigator (PI) and those involved at the clinical sites will note any side effects that subjects report. Occasionally, an ultra-concerned clinical investigator may turn up a problem that isn't one.

I recall a woman who developed a rash during clinical trials of a medication. Later, researchers determined that her caregiver had caused the rash by applying skin cream to her. The rash, however, continued to appear as a side effect of the drug. Despite the rash's mild severity and lack of connection to the medication, it indicated the researcher's strict adherence to protocol records.

Over the past several years, the discovery and prescribing of weight loss drugs (usually GLP-1) have been noted to have some mild side effects, and several studies have indicated what to expect in terms of side effects. Gut bacterial action causes bad breath (Ozempic breath), but it was easily manageable, provided the healthcare prescriber also examined any dental problems.

The Potential Risks

In another study, semaglutide was associated with a prevalence of nausea (44.10%), vomiting (24.58%), and gastroesophageal reflux disease (GERD) (6.28%) in obese individuals.

However, researchers are now expressing additional concerns about side effects that have emerged after tens of thousands of people have used these medications. How do these drugs work, and what are they noting?

By stimulating the body to create more insulin, these drugs decrease blood sugar levels. They also slow food's passage through the stomach and lessen the sugar released into the bloodstream. When the digestive process is delayed, patients experience prolonged feelings of fullness, which can reduce their caloric intake and lead to weight loss. The action of the drugs would seem beneficial, especially for those who need to control their blood sugar levels and their weight.

But there was an increased risk, however, of gastrointestinal disorders, hypotension, syncope, arthritic disorders, nephrolithiasis, and interstitial nephritis associated with GLP-1RA use compared to usual care.

Researchers also followed more than 200,000 diabetics taking GLP-1 meds and over 1.7 million diabetics using other medications to decrease blood sugar for around 3.5 years. The study did find that using GLP-1 was not without its hazards. They found these medications were associated with an increased risk of 146% of pancreatitis and 11% of arthritis. But most of the study's participants were white men in their 60s and 70s with US VA ties. Such a sample would not necessarily provide the most robust results, and future studies need to be much more diverse in the population studied.

The Vanity Factor

Aside from any physical effects, there is also something women especially might be concerned about: *Ozempic face.* A New York dermatologist came up with this term. It means that losing weight can make your face look older because of the tissue that is being lost. The fact that videos describing it have received millions of views indicates the extent of concern.

But when it comes to treating type 2 diabetes, the GLP-1 RA family provides positive benefits. In addition to a favorable impact on weight and a low risk of hypoglycemia, all medicines in the class have shown substantial reductions in A1C.

Despite some noted adverse side effects, the medications have proven beneficial to a significant number of users. However, we must carefully weigh the benefits and risks, and the Ozempic face should not be a negative factor when considering health-related issues.

Chapter 18: Who Needs Homework or Education, Anyway?

Take yourself back to your beginning school years, and what one feature of your schooling stands out? I'll bet it's all that homework that you were given and that your parents insisted you complete before you could go out to play or even go to bed at night. People viewed homework as the key to success in both school and life. Didn't do your homework? Well, that called for some sort of punishment or denial of privileges or whatever your cultural imperatives demanded for the surly child who would surely end up in the gutter if not for homework completion.

Ah, yes, homework provided the key to success in life, and, like any medication you would take for an ailment, it was the answer to all of life's future troubles and ills. It could, in the long run, help you pay for your medical bills. Imagine that.

Now, much to the chagrin of those of us who toiled through countless, numbing hours of saying our times tables aloud or persistently memorizing innumerable stanzas of impossible poems, the golden standard is being called into question. Wasn't memorizing "Oh, Captain, My Captain" worth all that time and effort at home and in class? How could that be? How could we question and view homework, something we held dear and sacred, as inessential?

Surely, it must be some kind of a pseudo-intellectual plot to keep our kids in underpaid, temporary jobs for the rest of their existence. Would the lack of homework lead to barely a subsistence lifestyle, no chicken in every pot, no car in the garage of our American-dream home, and dismal weeks in sweltering heat with no AC and no vacation? OMG, we are on the verge of something terrible—a world without homework. No, no, say it's not so.

For me, I think we really have to do what some researchers are now doing—study the research that has been done on homework and everything else and see how it relates to success in school. Avoid relying on the media for information, as it may distort the original findings. Actually, this little bit of ferreting out the truth in research is quite worthwhile.

For one thing, we make the assumption that doing homework actually has a beneficial effect on school performance, test scores, and success in college. Not so fast. Just asking how much time a kid spends on doing homework and how well they do in school may be insufficient to show anything. You should consider the other factors, like the homework's quality and its purpose for the child and the test.

Do national tests serve any purpose beyond providing reassurance that we are addressing our educational needs in this country? Or that we're concerned about the quality of our teachers? I don't think so. They may just be another way to fire teachers so they can't get tenure, a pension, or benefits, or any other perk that equals how much we spend on education. And we do want to educate our kids, don't we?

But what type of "education" we provide is a wholly different thing. Is education brainwashing or intellectual development? Do we want to raise a generation of thinkers and those who will question in the service of advancing knowledge or obedient pencil-pushers who will follow orders and be content with their sorry lot in life? We go from the inspired to the nefarious. Who is responsible for shaping this national mindset? Is it the product of true educators or those in the service of subservient mediocrity?

The key, of course, lies in who funds education and who promotes an agenda for the future. Eloquence used to support either side must always be carefully considered because, like in advertising, words can cause harm. Children and future generations will bear the brunt of the damage. Hark back to the 30s and listen to Orson Welles' voice of Lamont Cranston, "What evil lurks in the hearts of men? The Shadow knows."

Obviously, dear old Lamont was a seeker of truth and goodness, and boy, could we use him now. A well-placed political friend often attaches goodness and truth to a political donation or school board appointment. The school board, after all, is the stepping stone to higher political office, as we all know, so it's not necessarily a hotbed of people with a strong pedagogic bent. It's building a power base for the comers.

What do they say about good intentions? Yes, they pave the way to Hell, but I'm not that cynical. I do, however, believe that everything that seems like a noble intention isn't necessarily infused with that bit of fine morality. Remember, my friend, that words hold immense power and can serve a multitude of purposes. Therefore, pay attention to what is being said, but avoid consuming it in its entirety. Doing that can result in intellectual death.

One of the reasons I think national tests are thinly disguised as measures of something other than supposed good intentions is that the kids have been taught to train for them. This approach contradicts the principles of authentic education. Training for tests isn't the same as training for an athletic competition. When you train for the physical test, you build muscle, reaction time, and short-term goal planning and you have a very definite set of skills you need to develop. Training to take a specific test does nothing but hammer in rote memory without any consideration to questioning concepts. You absorb the information in its entirety, leaving no room for further inquiry. No questioning allowed. The true test of an education isn't just how well you can do a math problem, but how you can conceptualize how to address a problem that doesn't fit into a specific test-prep scheme your teachers have been doggedly running you through.

If tests were such good predictors of success in school and if even grades were such good predictors, why are more and more universities giving less weight to them on admissions criteria? Well, it seems that the SAT, GRE, MAT, or any other test really isn't a very good measure of anything other than a student's ability to take a test. Being good at test taking doesn't mean you are good at anything else and may indicate a rather rigid approach to education in general.

Visions of lockstepping kids are now dancing through my head as I see virtual and real teachers forcing compliance on kids who are becoming numb to the whole educational experience. Where's the joy, the adventure of learning, the questions that seem to have no answers, and are the latter okay to ask? Please, save the kids from this educational ghetto we're creating in the name of "standards." Could this be the cause of the surge in homeschooling among children? While this approach has its challenges, it can also nurture the budding intellects of children, ultimately benefiting everyone on this planet.

A non-profit think tank focused on the entire area of education and how best to provide it for everyone (not just kids at this point) would seem to pursue excellence as its goal. Many more people in this country would benefit from an education outside the school setting, but those who seek to fatten their bottom line seem to be the prime target, not the neuronal circuits of "learners." Don't you find that word a bit off-putting?

Okay, don't call them students or consumers, but is "learners" code for the newest entities on the block who want to gobble up all the educational funding (student loans included) without providing quality education at little to no cost? For me, I'm all for MOOCs (Massive Open Online Courses), but I'm concerned about those people who don't have access to computers or Internet access in their homes. These are the students I want all of us to reach and help them pull themselves up, but will the bias allow us to do this charity work toward others? Where can older adults, seniors, and children from low-income homes find free or inexpensive resources? There are sites.

Unfortunately, One Laptop per Child targets the "developing world," but does that encompass the United States? The Wiki article referenced two sites. But we do have a very real and very glaring need for free or extremely cheap computers for kids in this country, and they should be including our poor kids and struggling adults. Laptops and superior educational programs need to become available free of charge, and local libraries can help with a loaner program of inexpensive laptops. But what about Internet access? Establishing a local broadband service at no cost is also necessary to serve communities. Who benefits? Labeling it a social welfare program is too foolish to even debate, as it benefits all of us. If the NFL (National Football League), which earns billions each year, can get listed as a non-taxable entity, what about our citizens in need who live on something near subsistence?

Yes, it's charity because I believe we should all be giving in this effort to help others, especially the elderly who seek help but can't find it and have no tools to help them. Abe Lincoln may have made it in a log cabin with an oil lamp and books, but in today's world we shouldn't be looking back but forward in terms of technology and how we can help. How much of the US lacks Internet access? What parts of the country lack Internet access, and what is the job outlook like in those areas for anyone trying to earn a living wage? Do a little searching.

There are reasons people are denied this access, just as certain communities are denied bus routes. This situation is part of a plan that does not align with the values of caring for others. We should act based on what is right, but where can we find that sense of rightness in relation to education for everyone? Is there a genuine education that is accessible to everyone, regardless of their identity or location?

I think of the words of Hillel, "*...if I am but for myself, And if I am only for myself, then what am I...*"

Chapter 19: Where Have All the Sidewalks Gone?

Environments and ecology are major concerns for all of us, not just today, but for the past 60 years, when we began to hear teachers talk about it. Then, it was a new idea, a new challenge, and we didn't quite know where it would lead us. But now we are beginning to appreciate how that butterfly in the forest and its fluttering wings have such great meaning for the entire planet. Butterflies, in fact, are becoming an aspect of natural beauty that, like the honeybees, are few and far between thanks to our wonderful pest controllers.

Jane Jacobs sounded the bell of warning about our cities and what we needed to preserve in order to remain a cohesive and wonderful conglomerate society. She knew what we would lose if only one bit of a mundane feature of our cities was lost, and it was the sidewalks.

The portion from her book, "The Life and Death of Great American Cities," which made a compelling case for sidewalks, reads:

"A city sidewalk by itself is nothing. It is an abstraction. It means something only in conjunction with the buildings and other uses that border it, or border other sidewalks very near it. The same might be said of streets, in the sense that they serve other purposes besides carrying wheeled traffic in their middles. Streets and their sidewalks, the main public places of a city, are its most vital organs. Think of a city, and what comes to mind? Its streets. If a city's streets look interesting, the city looks interesting; if they look dull, the city looks dull."

If sidewalks form the vital organs of a city, great or not, what does the lack of them mean to us? Where have Americans fled in the past 50 years? They've scurried from the cities to escape to the wooded glens and welcoming hills with trim lawns we call suburbia. It is here that, theoretically, children can be raised in comfort and safety. It was part of the American dream, but we must now assess what we lost and gained.

Writing primarily, I presume, about her beloved New York City's Greenwich Village area and deriving much of her inspiration from it, she wasn't the only one thinking about the vital connections sidewalks create. An article in The Austin Chronicle made a powerful statement about sidewalks where it indicates:

"Residents and visitors may walk around easily within their confines, but doing something as simple as crossing neighboring streets may still be impossible. Austin becomes a chain of islands of walkability, with oceans of dirt trails and dangerous multi-lane asphalt between them."

The utility of sidewalks for pedestrian flow and interaction is obvious, and the tenor of a neighborhood can quickly be gauged by either the condition and availability of its sidewalks or the lack of them. Where there are no sidewalks present, it would seem pedestrians are not welcomed, or sidewalks serve only as afterthoughts for the residents and city management.

Where sidewalks are welcoming, they encourage interaction, casual exercise and neighborhood involvement through the many observers who use them. They are not, therefore, mere forebears of the era of the horseless carriages but a reminder that we are all connected, and to maintain these connections, we must plan our cities and villages diligently to preserve that which is good and necessary.

Walking down a street with a child, hand-in-hand, is far more enriching than strapping them into the back seat of your SUV. Research has proven that tactile interactions are vital for human growth potential in both social and intellectual aspects. Spending those quiet moments can be more precious and engaging than you might think. Have you tried it lately, or is it impossible to do where you live?

Should you have been fortunate enough to grow up, or spend the first formative years of your life, in an area where sidewalks were a part of the landscape, think back to what they meant in your life. You probably just took it for granted and never realized how vital this simple bit of footpath was in your life.

Columbia, Maryland planners began to realize that a city plan with sidewalk access to most of it could be one of the most important enhancements for its citizens. The idea was in direct opposition to the stark and isolated subdivision community design then so prevalent. The year 1947 saw the rise of a portion of the plan by the powerful New York City mogul, Robert Moses, for the development of Long Island, and with it came Levittown, NY.

Levittown would be one of many such communities built around the country as the idea was cloned time and time again. The result led to dull, tree-stripped neighborhood destruction, not development in the true sense of the word. Neighbors became more like isolated tenants in cookie-cutter houses than friends.

Moses may have been seen as a force for development and foresight, but he destroyed the small neighborhood concept that kept communities vibrant and ripped through them with concrete highways leading to developers' money pots. Neighborhoods, especially those in lower-income areas, were fractured and separated by high walls supporting the roadways, and the communities withered. He would have destroyed downtown Manhattan had his plans not been thwarted.

Replacing small shops, bustling sidewalks and friendly neighbor encounters was quite an effortless task for Moses and his planners. They built "projects" that seemed "modern" but were unsafe and unfriendly brick prisons for those who couldn't afford to move to the suburbs. The less fortunate were left in buildings that afforded a criminal element easy access in unlighted hallways and elevators that failed to work. The design concept plans really didn't portray what would follow, where little would be dedicated to trees and small shops. The buildings would abut highways or less desirable areas. Ghettos were created.

Where have all the sidewalks gone? We have to not only wonder but begin to concern ourselves with a return to sidewalks where teens don't have to get into cars to drive miles to friends' homes. A trip to the store, too, shouldn't require an SUV.

Chapter 20: Death and the Cancer Screen Not Performed

Today's New York Times has a timely and important article by the respected science writer Jane Brody, a woman with an advanced science degree and a breast cancer survivor. I always read her articles because they are chock-full of information I want and need about health, the environment and all things science/life related. But today's on whether or not people should continue to get cancer screenings for various illnesses, even those not prone to the cancer, caught my eye. Something has been burning inside my brain for three years now, and it's time for it to come out, and the Brody article did it.

One of my beloved sisters was a model of self-care in terms of her health. She went for her yearly physical and her yearly mammogram, saw the dermatologist for any suspicious skin spots, and exercised daily. No slouch, she rode a bike, helped repair her relatives' homes, painted, loved all the neighborhood kids, and was a ready friend and confidante when someone needed one. Honest, a straight arrow and always ready to fight for the underdog, she was a champion for all of us.

When we heard she had fallen suddenly at her home and was taken to the hospital, all of us were shocked. She'd never been hospitalized, except for the birth of her children, had no illnesses and only suffered from allergies. That's all we knew, but there was a dark and dangerous thing taking over her life in a manner that shouldn't have happened.

Smoking helps people cope with stress and bouts of anxiety in many situations, and years ago it was no big deal to smoke. Homes were readily furnished with plenty of ashtrays, and cigarettes were everywhere. Teens wanted to smoke. People in films smoked somewhat excessively, and famous people all had cigarettes in hand. Look at *Edward R. Murrow, John Wayne, Steve McQueen, Bette Davis and Walter Cronkite*. They all smoked.

How does smoking help? Nicotine is a natural substance in our body's nervous system, and, in fact, there are special receptors for it in the spinal cord. So it serves a natural purpose, but not when teamed up with the ingredients in cigarettes that make them remain lit or light faster or whatever. Lots of additives to keep those little sticks burning.

Actually, there are benefits from those receptors, but we don't really have to add to their workload by inhaling cigarette smoke. They work just fine as they are.

Cigarettes, therefore, were ways to introduce extra nicotine into our bodies, and they did quell anxiety to a degree. These innocent white sticks were much like anti-anxiety meds but without the need for a prescription. Alcohol serves much the same purpose for some people, and that's part of the process that leads to addiction. The addiction to cigarettes, I've read, is as strong as that for heroin.

Social situations where the stress may have been ramped up were always ones where cigarettes were plentiful. They added to our level of comfort and gave us something to do when we found our hands were uncomfortably hanging at our sides. Behavioral cues only helped reinforce smoking in more situations, and it became natural to light up their first smoke before they got out of bed in the morning.

My sister was a smoker for over 40 years until family members, concerned about the dangers of smoking, managed to help her rid herself of the "cancer sticks," as we called them. She tried more than once, and she did succeed. For over 20 years she hadn't smoked. It didn't matter because the fire inside had been lit, and it remained a burning, growing ember no one suspected was there.

After the fall, she was in the hospital for a quick exam. The ER physician ordered x-rays, and they, according to him, showed nothing. She and her husband went back home, where her pain intensified. Back to another hospital, where they found a fracture of the hip, which would require surgery. The first ER physician had missed the fracture. While there for this evaluation, her family physician passed by and asked, "Why are you here? You're never sick."

Never sick because he never did one thing that a smoker with a long history of smoking requires: an occasional x-ray of the lungs. He never did one for her annual exam even though he had been seeing her for over 30 years and knew she had been a smoker. Not one lung x-ray with all those mammograms, colonoscopies and skin exams. Not one.

Yes, they had found some benign polyps on her colonoscopy one year, but it was nothing to be worried about. Our mother died of colon cancer, but they told her she was fine. And she believed them because they were the healers and she was only a patient with a family history of cancers of many types: colon, skin, breast, bone and eye. Her family physician knew of this history.

The hip surgery and the pre-surgical medical workup revealed extensive, metastatic cancer of the lung, bone and perhaps brain. Despite what she had been told, and I have to wonder how much she was told, she decided to have the hip surgery because, as she said, "I won't be able to walk if I don't have it." Did anyone tell her the gravity of the diagnosis and that she wouldn't have more than two months to walk with her current diagnosis?

After the surgery, she went to rehab, and they did more CAT scans, and then they wanted to do chemotherapy when the full extent of the illness hit her with one of those "talks" about care. "*I'm going to heaven,*" she said with an audible choke in her throat and stopped our conversation dead.

She refused the chemo, which would have had her sick as a dog for every remaining day of her life. And the days remaining, even with the therapy, would be short indeed. Home was where she wanted to be, and that's where she went with her pain medication and the hospice care they provided.

No longer would I have my sister as I had known her. Drugged almost to the point of being unconscious, she carried on and was carefully dressed for each of my visits until she could no longer even sit up when I came. Two months after the diagnosis, she died in the care of a family member who is a nurse. She'd stopped eating and could barely take a sip of tea, and then she slipped away quietly in the early morning hours.

Not one x-ray with all those other exams. I'm not advocating for x-rays because we know they're not totally safe (as isn't extensive plane travel or dental x-rays). But I am advocating for more care on the part of people who have knowledge of family and personal history—family physicians. One x-ray may have saved her life, but we'll never know.

Chapter 21: Public Places and Private Spaces

Environmentalists aren't only passionate about preserving the wild places (always reminds me of Maurice Sendak when I say "wild") and the habitats of our planet's species. Those who march and collect and petition also have one other species besides the whales, the lions, the tiny fishes living in underground pools in the West, or the spectacular Monarch butterflies on a yearly trek to Mexico. These intrepid souls also want to save places for you, me, and generations to come.

A battle of sorts was started at least 50 years ago in New York City, where discrete, quiet, highly personal space was becoming a luxury, especially outside the overpriced and too tiny apartments offered at almost prohibitive rents.

Rent control was seen as one way to save the city for those who were born there, moved to work there, or were spending their final decade there in anything-but-glamorous living spaces. People filed lawsuits, engaged in shouting matches in the City Council chambers, and faced physical assaults and denials of their right to assemble. It was often brutish and certainly bordered on illegal. Money and funding of political campaigns seemed to be holding sway.

Greedy and unscrupulous landlords, under the subterfuge of "renovation," tore kitchen floors and bathroom fixtures out while the tenants were still in residence. Little was done as they went about their tenant-destruction plans. Ceilings fell down, water came from pipes, floors were unsafe and kitchens were unusable. All of this took place under the questionably watchful eye of the building department charged with protecting the rights and the safety of New York City citizens. The protectors had been bought off. Some went to jail.

Bribes had been paid, and inspectors vigorously ignored exhortations to review the condition of apartments. The city's 311 line was of no use to tenants. Too many tenants were convinced, ultimately, that they had no rights and that there was no help for them. Often they were elderly persons with disabilities or medical illnesses, those who spoke little English, or those who had no financial means to engage attorneys to work on their behalf.

Intolerable? Surely, but what about the other spaces that would have been denied to a different group of citizens who had remained silent as others suffered? The pace of luxury real estate construction is at dizzying heights as even the most undesirable neighborhoods in rat-infested areas are turned into million-dollar condos for the ultra-wealthy and, often, foreign investors who never live there.

The cherry on top of the cake is the construction of two entrances to at least one luxury building: one for the rich and the other the "poor" door. The latter was necessitated as developers were required to provide affordable housing for the middle class in these new buildings. It was the architectural equivalent of "in your face" action. Yet another example of the two- (or three-) class society that is developing in New York City.

One response to the overdevelopment of Manhattan, and now Brooklyn, was an attempt by the city mothers and fathers, who convinced some architects that space was needed. The spaces were to be little places where the work-weary citizens could escape the go-go-go pace of work for at least a half-hour. They were lovely, relatively quiet and, where possible, sunlit. They were known as "pocket parks." The parks in New York City were scattered in tiny, discrete spots much like pleasant coves in a turbulent sea. The ones I saw were primarily on the East Side, the area of Manhattan that is most desirable.

The question now is whether or not even these pocket parks will withstand the sledgehammers and backhoes of the developers who appear to be becoming ever more avaricious in their quest to build yet higher condos for the billionaires of the world. An interesting graph points out how the "reach for the sky" mania has progressed in this premiere city.

In fact, even those who covet their Louboutin and Jimmy Choo shoes are being affected. Wonder if Carrie Bradshaw of "Sex and the City" fame would still be able to afford the rent if she hadn't married Mr. Big.

One would think that the middle-class working stiffs would be the only group grousing about rents, overcrowded streets, lack of privacy and that one commodity becoming so scarce—actual sunlight on the streets. Yes, the buildings are designed with little regard to how they reflect unwanted, often eye-irritating light into apartment windows while denying it to the streets below. The skyscrapers even present dangers when snowstorms leave icy slabs on their slanted roofs and streets must be closed to traffic and pedestrians alike.

Now it's the turn of the wealthy who see themselves as only millionaires or at least "comfortable" in a world peopled by billionaires. Yes, poor things, they have their travails due to the encroaching real estate boom. They've even begun to protest what they see as a sense of a neighborhood being lost in the shadow of the "billionaire tower" that is proposed to be built. Nice to know they're beginning to see what others have suffered through for the last several decades.

When studio apartment dwellers are offered $1M to vacate, you know there's money to be had. Wonder what they offered the people who lived in the neighborhoods ripped up by the building of the Cross-Bronx Expressway. I'll bet it wasn't one-tenth of that, and it was just get out because your home is being demolished.

Even New York City's mayor is becoming restive when it comes to city space for people. His predecessor, Michael Bloomberg, a multi-billionaire in his own right, turned a portion of Broadway into an open-air sitting park that quickly became filled with people in cartoon-character outfits posing for photos (for a fee) with tourists. The biggest push for the mayor came when women "clothed" in little more than body paint pranced onto the scene with their male "protectors," who collected the fees. The mayor's response? Rip it all up and be done with it.

Does it seem reasonable to deny the many because of the actions of the few? After all, Mayor, we've had The Naked Cowboy on Broadway for many years. I once met him in a garage at the end of his "shift," and he graciously posed for a free photo. Nice guy, I must say.

Precious little space is available in New York City, and what is there is evaporating like the glaciers. While we cannot immediately take action to preserve the glaciers, certainly solutions for the city are not without an agreeable compromise.

Quality of life is a major consideration not just in terms of our physical condition but also in terms of the places where we choose to live. Active participation of all in maintaining these quiet, open and not wild places is for all of us, not just the well-heeled.

But Manhattan is headed in that direction, especially when you hear that one condo recently sold for $100.5M. The owner won't have to worry about open space because there's nothing as high as the tower in which he/she lives. The island of Manhattan lies at their feet, carpeted by the less fortunate.

Chapter 22: Recipe for Creating Monsters

Mary Wollstonecraft Shelley, in a contest meant to pass time in a mountain cabin while on a winter vacation, created one of our most recognizable monsters, Frankenstein. But, if you read the story carefully, you will find the psychology that is hidden from the casual reader.

It's not a story of evil and monsters but of brutish behavior, intolerance and rampant fear of the different. We can find it in our own culture today, but it's not always so obvious until we begin cataloging the headlines that indicate murder, aggression toward others, cruelty toward children and ordinary citizens. The stories might stand as signposts for cause-and-effect actions today as it may have during the 19th century. But Shelley may not have meant to do other than be creative.

The media these days is rife with articles and TV news stories about violence in all forms—against adults, children and animals. Do we live in a violent age, and if we do, what can we do to remediate this and bring back some civility and sense? Look at some of the things that research has told us contribute to the making of violent individuals who are not necessarily psychotic but bent on actions that will result in headlines to give them some measure of notoriety.

However, even the very research on which we psychologists depend for extending our knowledge in our field is now under question. A recent effort on the part of 250 psychologists, who reviewed research in 100 published psychology papers and who tried to replicate the results, came back with rather dismal results. Only 36% had meaningful results, and, unbelievably, an astounding 80% of the original researchers had overstated their findings. Pretty discouraging for all of us. If we can't depend on scientific data regarding our work, what is there left for us?

Do we now have to begin wearing Carnac hats and divining the contents of envelopes or some other sort of circus act?

First, before we look at some research we believe is helpful, a few words about the latest sensation in social media. Social media have been a boon to all of us, and no one can deny that, but they also bear a heavy responsibility in specific circumstances, such as the on-camera murder of two journalists in Virginia on August 26, 2015. It was the ultimate in reality TV, to which too many have become addicted. And it spread like wildfire across the globe thanks, again, to social media outlets like YouTube and Facebook.

True, social media took the footage down quickly, but there was no way it hadn't already been grabbed by thousands or millions of computers. Just what directory would you use for something like that, or would you create a special one? The grisly scene will live on, and with it the man who committed the crime, as two innocent people went about their job filming an interview about a business event.

The New York Times columnist, Farhad Manjoo, wrote, "*The horror was the dawning realization, as the video spread across the networks, that the killer had anticipated the moves—that he had been counting on the mechanics of these services and our inability to resist passing on what he had posted.*" It was the internet age's example of drivers slowing down to get a better look at a horrific auto accident on the highway. The bloodier, the better, as the drivers shook their heads but scoped in nevertheless.

For the moment, let's accept that social media did the right thing in taking the footage down. But let's not accept that The New York Daily News, after bearing the brunt of some pretty serious media ostracization for printing a video grab of the killing, the next day ran the actual video on its website.

Is that like thumbing your nose at those who questioned the News' type of journalism? I don't think people take the newspaper very seriously anyway, so this type of juvenile response was to be expected from its editorial staff. It seems clearly in the vein of yellow journalism and sensationalism for which they are known.

No one really needs to lay out a plan or recipe for creating a "monster" with a predisposition to violence. Pretty much we know that they feel either wronged, neglected, or underappreciated or want to desperately make someone else feel as badly as they do.

It may begin in early childhood, and when it does, and that's pretty much the idea, it has plenty of time to develop. Fruition comes with growth, strength and the ability to plan actions or, often, to just let the fuse burn full tilt. When it does the latter, the explosion can be totally unanticipated but a reason for fear now and in the future. The stage has been set unless there's speedy intervention.

One thing child psychologists or developmental psychologists agree on is that a lack of structure, predictability and adherence to a reasonable, responsible and firm set of rules of behavior are required for normal development. Lacking in one or more of these may bring on a sense of resentment and a belief that rules are never to be understood or followed because the rules and the consequences are always changing.

Psychologists call it a typical double-bind situation; sometimes an action is okay, and other times, it means punishment. There's never any certainty about the end result, so why not try to get away with something? You never know; you might just slip by without any consequences.

The current state of our understanding of human behavior or misbehavior isn't all that great. The research is still going on, and only recently did one medical investigator discover that the brain has a system totally unknown before: its own lymphatic system. How could it have been missed?

The discovery may not mean very much to you, but to scientists it is astounding and may open research in areas never even considered possible when it came to the brain and its functioning or vulnerability to disease. Think what it may mean to the healing or prevention of neurological diseases. Truly wonderful surprises are yet to come.

Ask yourself how many things are missed; we take it for granted that we've already discovered all there is. Look for the unexpected. Isn't that how a new bone was discovered within the past two years? Shouldn't we have gotten all of those bones right before now? Obviously, the answer is no, we hadn't and there's more to be discovered.

The brain has not given up all its secrets, and it jealously guards them from us, revealing itself only to those with tenacious curiosity, those who think outside the box and refuse current orthodoxy. Isn't that what's happening in Alzheimer's research now? Aren't they beginning to question that billion-dollar quest for the amyloid plaque theory that they all thought was going to be the answer to our prayers?

What about autism and schizophrenia? Didn't they think it was all the mother's or the parents' fault when a child developed either? Now we know autism begins in the womb, and so may schizophrenia. The parents are the only ones that professionals targeted because the pros didn't know any better, and they, too, went along with the popular thinking of the day.

The thinking now is that autism may actually be a form of creativity. In some cases, we should stop thinking of it as a disorder and begin seeing it as a specific talent or gift. How about that way of thinking to turn things around?

For many decades, professionals studying hypnosis found that children appeared to be the best subjects. What was the reason? They proposed it's because children have not been cut off from their imagination and creativity by the rules imposed in adulthood. A return to some of the things that we call "childish" may be in our best interests, and play has become a new area of research. What was childhood known for? How about a sense of freedom from adult rules of thinking? All of those "why?" questions were good ones, and we shouldn't think we have the answers.

Can you think of something more anomalous than telling an adult that they need to learn to play? If you did that, they'd think you'd been eating some of those amazing little candies or treats they make in Colorado.

How does any of this relate to making monsters? Simply put, we make monsters through our own diligent efforts to marginalize, discriminate against and loathe individuals who are different. We impose rules that cannot be followed, engage in intolerant behaviors ourselves, and refuse to look for the good. We also cut off our own explorations into the "whys" of some behaviors to find the "what can we do" responses that will help.

The state of our current ignorance in too much is so shocking that it defies even considering. Perhaps it's easier to go on in a dogmatic fashion, believing what we've been told is the "truth" about too much and too many. I believe that we can't find answers because we haven't even asked the questions yet, and we don't even know how to do that.

For once, let's give a cheer for those who dare to look for answers that others have said have already been found. Those who refuse to accept the current medical theology instead brave new pathways to find the hidden treasure we deny exists.

Chapter 23:
The Nose May Determine Why Your Cognition Declines

Working on a national protocol for a new medication for Alzheimer's disease allowed me an opportunity to understand some of the pathology involved. Many decades ago, researchers tested a specific aspect of cognitive decline: the sense of smell.

Prior research had indicated a direct connection between the loss of a sense of smell and the incipient appearance of symptoms of Alzheimer's disease. Many years later, researchers are beginning to explore that connection more vigorously since it may be more fruitful than we ever anticipated.

Memory, cognitive abilities, and brain function can all decline to different degrees as people age, especially around middle age. Notably, dementia and other age-related cognitive decline disorders have been on the rise for several years. Of course, when seeking causes for something such as a neurodegenerative disorder, we immediately look at the environment, diet, and lifestyle, but how many of us look to a person's sense of smell?

Neurodegenerative illnesses are now commonly linked to a diminished sense of smell. While not all individuals with Alzheimer's, Parkinson's, Huntington's, or schizophrenia may experience olfactory abnormalities, these conditions can manifest in certain patients. It is unclear if these symptoms are a result of the disease itself or if they are caused by a malfunctioning olfactory system that promotes neuronal death in many brain locations through circuit changes. Finding olfactory receptors in non-sensory regions of the brain is another component of the olfactory pathway to neurodegenerative disorders.

The number of people diagnosed with dementia is projected to rise from 55 million in 2019 to approximately 139 million by 2050, according to estimates. Therefore, it is critically important to understand what causes cognitive decline and how to identify the early symptoms of dementia so that therapeutic measures can be planned appropriately.

Olfaction, the sense of smell, is related to multiple areas within the central nervous system, many of which are directly related to the development of psychiatric illnesses, neurogenic disorders such as Parkinson's, and even schizophrenia. Studies have indicated that over 139 conditions are in some way related to a sense of smell, including MS, ALS, and other cognitive dysfunction disorders. Other, less understood relationships between smell and a physical disorder include cardiovascular disease, arthritis, and polycystic ovary syndrome. All of these disorders point to the wide range of associations between scent receptors in the body and physical or mental disturbances.

During the pandemic, when COVID-19 was running throughout the United States, people began to understand that a loss of a sense of smell was one of the signs that they may have become infected. In fact, in Alzheimer's research, we have found that smell is one of the first senses affected. In COVID-19, this loss of a sense of smell pointed to the virus having more of an ability to damage our nervous system. We now know that COVID is much more of a serious, probably neurologic infection than previously thought, and that it can linger for a long time. In Alzheimer's, smell pointed to neurologic damage that had already begun, and of which researchers were aware.

In fact, the physical location of our sense of smell and its relationship to other aspects of our lives is paramount. Opposite to sounds, odors travel directly to the olfactory bulb embedded in the forebrain. The bulb is associated with numerous brain regions that play a role in emotional regulation, decision-making, memory, and learning.

While neurological injury certainly accounts for some olfactory impairment, newer studies indicate that a loss of smell may be a contributing component to our reduced total lifespan. This is a scary thought; we would do anything to prolong our lives. We exercise, we watch our diet, and we try to maintain healthy, social relationships, so why not pay some attention to our sense of smell?

Training Our Sense of Smell

Observing the widespread utilization of smell receptors has pointed researchers to a new appreciation of an intriguing and somewhat unusual idea regarding smell and cognition training.

Can we train ourselves in some way to affect the health or preserve the utility of our scent receptors? In other words, is smell a trainable human ability? Undoubtedly, animals have far greater abilities to detect scents outside of human capacity. Still, we are not talking about approaching that level of sensitivity but merely enhancing what we have now.

If we can train our sense of smell, we can protect and preserve our cognition. It sounds rather unusual, or if you prefer, bizarre, but that is what is being considered now. But the current research goes even further, indicating that we may be able to repair or revive smell receptors that may have gone dormant through our aging process. We know that the sense of smell seems to diminish with age, but now there is new hope for our smell receptors.

Research has surged because "smell training" may revive this dormant sense and improve cognitive abilities. Evidence from studies points to the possibility that it can. The more we utilize our sense of smell, the more powerful it becomes, like a muscle.

Could we achieve favorable results in scent training by doing more than just following our noses? Many commercially available smell-training programs seek to achieve that. In most cases, the instructions for using the kits call for the user to spend a few minutes daily sniffing a blend of fragrant compounds, including clove, eucalyptus, rose, and lemon, for a few weeks or months.

Experiments have shown heightened sensitivity to odors with a negligible time commitment. Be patient. For instance, a study indicated that individuals with post-infectious olfactory dysfunction showed substantial recovery in 70% of cases when treated for 56 weeks, compared to 58% when trained for 15 weeks.

While the user sleeps, a partially available device releases 40 distinct aromas. Results showed a 226% improvement in verbal memory following six months of nightly usage in a short experiment that examined an early version on 43 individuals aged 60 to 85. Of course, such a small sample needs to be considered carefully and much larger. We need larger samples to achieve professional acceptance and determine whether this training is practical.

Chapter 24: Stress Is the Brain Drain Robbing You of Everything

B ooks are a buzz with stress, but how many of us take it to heart and how can we begin to gain power over it and help ourselves in the process?

During test preparation, you sit down to study, yet your mind remains completely empty. You have lost your locker combination for the third time this week, but you used it every day during the previous months. This experience matches yours while you maintain a normal mental state. The scientific term for brain drain is stress-induced cognitive impairment.

Your Brain on Stress: What's Really Happening?

Brain cells transform when stress occurs because your mental fog becomes real. Stanford University research demonstrates that excessive stress triggers your brain to produce cortisol in large amounts, which should serve emergency purposes, but develops toxicity through prolonged presence. The prolonged activation of cortisol functions as a fire alarm that becomes ignored yet continues to harm your hearing ability.

The hippocampus experiences shrinkage when stress persists according to Dr. Robert Sapolsky's Stanford research because this brain area controls memory and learning functions. Your amygdala enlarges due to stress so you become more sensitive to perceiving threats in your environment. You might think of it as the smoke detector in your brain alerting you when you burn toast yet your fire extinguisher gradually reduces in size with time. A good visual to keep in mind here.

Being overwhelmed represents only a portion of this problem. The research conducted at Harvard Medical School demonstrates that stress impairs your brain's working memory function which enables information manipulation. Working memory functions become impaired during exam week when students struggle to understand simple math problems and they must read the same paragraph multiple times without retaining any information. Does that sound familiar?

The Hidden Costs: What Stress Steals From You

Chronic stress produces multiple negative effects which reach further than students' test performance. Research conducted at the University of California Berkeley demonstrated how stress damages neuroplasticity which represents the brain's ability to create new neural pathways. Your brain struggles to remember information, but the real challenge lies in losing your efficient learning capacity.

Stress leads to deterioration of both sleep quality and creativity levels and destroys social relationships. Sleep Medicine Reviews published research showing that stressed students experience disrupted sleep patterns even though they obtain sufficient rest. What's more, sleep problems create additional stress, which creates an enduring cycle of stress that proves challenging to interrupt.

Stress has the most alarming effect on how people make decisions. Research conducted at MIT showed chronic stress drives the brain to perform automatic responses instead of contemplative decision-making. Students who experience stress make bad decisions regarding their time use, relationships, and their health because their brains function automatically.

The conventional advice about stress management appears both unhelpful and unrealistic to many people. The following science-based weekly planning system exists to shield your brain from excessive stress while providing an alternative to "just relax" advice.

Monday: Micro-Recovery Mapping

Dedicate 10 minutes on Monday to identify three daily "micro-recovery" intervals which should be your focus rather than creating a weekly plan. Spend 2–3 minutes performing activities which stimulate your parasympathetic nervous system through deep breathing progressive muscle relaxation or viewing nature pictures. According to University of Melbourne research this nature image viewing decreases cortisol in 40 seconds. Considering that short length of time, this is very impressive and very useful.

Tuesday: Task Batching by Energy Type

Organize your tasks into groups according to mental energy requirements instead of following traditional subject-based organization. Your natural peak hours should be dedicated to creative thinking tasks which include writing essays and brainstorming yet processing tasks such as note organization and fact-checking should be done when your energy levels are lower.

Wednesday: Worry Window Scheduling

Dedicate 15 minutes daily to concern yourself with every worry that exists in your mind. List every concern, no matter how insignificant it seems. Tell yourself that you will handle everything during your designated worry period whenever worries arise throughout the day. The worry postponement method has proven to lower anxiety levels by 25% in clinical trials.

Thursday: Social Connection Calibration

Plan one essential social activity that excludes school-related work and stress. The time should be spent on authentic family discussions or laughter with friends or animal interaction. Positive social connections, according to UCLA research, also decreases cortisol levels more effectively than many standard stress-reduction approaches.

Friday: Future Self Visualization

Set aside 5 minutes to picture yourself succeeding in reaching your weekend targets. The essential aspect here lies in visualizing the steps to reach your goal rather than focusing solely on the end result. You should picture yourself performing the tasks and handling minor challenges, along with feeling empowered. The mental contrasting method enhances both stress resistance and motivational power.

Saturday: Sensory Reset Day

Devote your attention to one sense throughout the entire day. Choose to fully experience the flavors of your food, actively listen to environmental noises, or feel various textures. The mindfulness practice helps both your nervous system reset and enhances your brain's focus abilities. You're not only handling stress, you are building your own power base to handle it in the future.

Sunday: Weekly Brain Dump and Celebration

Record everything you achieved throughout the week regardless of how insignificant your achievements seem. Often, we tend to dismiss many of these small achievements we have made; nothing is to be dismissed. Afterward create a list of your upcoming week's concerns. Write down one thing you discovered about your stress patterns and about yourself. Your brain needs this reflection time to process the week's events while preparing for upcoming difficulties.

The Science of Small Changes

Scientific studies show that regular minor changes lead to positive neuroplasticity, which enables your brain to develop new stress management capabilities. Research at the University of Wisconsin demonstrated that practicing micro-intervention activities led to observable brain structural modifications in participants over an eight-week period.

Remember that your brain operates as a protective mechanism to shield you from harm. Your mind exists to protect you, yet requires assistance to function optimally. You can recover your mental clarity and performance by understanding how stress impacts your thinking abilities while using targeted stress management techniques.

The mental fog you experience will pass because it remains temporary and you bear no responsibility for it and it is absolutely curable. Your brain demonstrates remarkable strength, while proper tools enable you to work together with it rather than fighting against each other.

Chapter 25: Beware of the Hidden Mental Health Threats in Your Food

New research is raising concerns about the mental health aspects of the foods that we eat and that we believe are perfectly safe.

Scientific studies show a link between ocean microplastics and mental health issues. While the mounting evidence is highly disturbing, our bodies are experiencing even more direct destruction.

Human brains contain up to 30 times more microplastics than livers or kidneys, a Nature Medicine study reveals. The microplastic concentration in the brains of dementia patients exceeded levels three to five times higher than those found in non-dementia patients. While this may seem shocking, consider that the overall brain microplastic content increased by 50% between 2016 and 2024. Should we simply disregard this increase, or do microplastics present a more significant issue that requires attention beyond just the oceans?

The Ultra-Processed Food Connection

The primary entry point for brain-invasive microplastics is found in ultra-processed foods, which account for more than half of the calories consumed by the average American daily. Instant noodles, packaged snacks, carbonated drinks, chicken nuggets, and many other convenient foods available in grocery stores represent ultra-processed foods.

These foods naturally contain microplastics because industrial processes and plastic packaging systems introduce them. Chicken nuggets have way more microplastics than chicken breast — like, 30 times more per gram! Three minutes of microwaving a plastic container results in the release of more than four million microplastic particles from one square centimeter of plastic material.

The Mental Health Crisis Connection

The mental health issues of depression and anxiety, worldwide, aren't coincidental. The rise of depression and anxiety symptoms appears to coincide with the growing consumption of ultra-processed foods in society. A substantial review of 10 million participants in a BMJ study demonstrated that people who consumed ultra-processed foods faced depression at 22% higher rates, anxiety at 48% higher rates, and sleep disturbances at 41% higher rates.

People who maintained their diet with nutrient-dense, unprocessed foods showed minimal instances of mental health problems.

The Ways Microplastics Harm the Brain

The ways through which microplastics may cause mental health damage exist in complex and disturbing combinations. Microplastics enter the brain by crossing the blood-brain barrier to interfere with nerve communication functions through multiple mechanisms.

Acetylcholine, alongside GABA and glutamate, exhibits changes in its brain chemical levels when microplastics interact with brain chemistry. These neurotransmitters also serve as targets for antidepressant and anti-anxiety medications.

Microplastics and nanoplastics can increase the risk of neuropsychiatric disorders by inducing oxidative stress in the brain, causing nerve cell damage, and influencing the functionality of neurotransmitters. Oxidative stress occurs when these particles generate free radicals that damage brain cells, which may also make neurons more susceptible to psychiatric disorders.

The plastic particles that contain endocrine-disrupting chemicals like BPA disrupt hormonal systems responsible for mood control and stress response.

The SMILES Study: Proof That Food Changes Work

The relationship between processed foods and mental health problems exists in reality beyond theory. The fundamental research in nutritional psychiatry known as the SMILES trial shows essential findings. Researchers studied sixty-seven participants with moderate to severe depression; half followed their standard diet, while the other half consumed unprocessed Mediterranean-style foods.

The research showed outstanding findings because 32% of patients in the dietary intervention group achieved depression remission during the 12-week study period, but only 8% of the control group succeeded. Dietary intervention enabled participants to eliminate 22 processed food items weekly, likely reducing their microplastic exposure.

Three Research-Backed Steps to Protect Your Mental Health

The present understanding of microplastics and mental health enables you to implement the following actionable steps starting today to minimize exposure and safeguard your brain health:

1. Dramatically Reduce Ultra-Processed Foods

To reduce your exposure, eliminate most packaged snacks, instant meals, processed meats, sugary drinks, and fast food. Your food choices should focus on fresh fruits and vegetables, lean proteins, whole grains, nuts, and legumes.

The single dietary modification addresses the most significant source of microplastic exposure through food while simultaneously boosting your nutritional intake. The SMILES study demonstrated that participants who switched to this new diet saw significant improvements in depression symptoms during twelve weeks.

Practical tip: Purchase fresh products by walking along the store perimeter instead of entering the center section, which contains processed foods. As someone who once participated in a supermarket design study, I know how foods are placed in the store to attempt to attract you to pick up specific items.

Some items are more difficult to reach, while others are readily placed where you will quickly toss them into your grocery basket without thought. Stores use what is known as "sore thumb displays" that stick out from the standard shelving to give them extra attention. The checkouts are similarly designed for maximum profit and consumer access.

Eliminate Plastic from Food Storage and Heating

Plastic containers should never be used to microwave food, and microwave-safe plastic wrap should always be avoided during heating. The best choice for food storage and reheating is to use glass or ceramic containers. Avoid consuming hot beverages in plastic cups or bottles.

The process of heating plastic results in the massive release of microplastics, which generates millions of particles during brief heating periods. The storage of food at room temperature inside plastic containers proves to be safer than any heated storage methods.

Practical tip: Buy a set of glass containers with secure lids for preparing meals and storing food.

Adopt a Mediterranean-Style Eating Pattern

Use your dietary choices to select foods with proven mental health benefits, such as fatty fish, olive oil, nuts, seeds, colorful vegetables, fruits, and whole grains. Would you like to know which types of fish are both healthier for you and more budget-friendly? Several inexpensive, fatty fish are also considered very healthy, particularly for heart health. These include sardines, mackerel, anchovies, and canned salmon. These fish are excellent sources of omega-3 fatty acids, which are essential for heart health.

This eating pattern naturally avoids processed foods while delivering maximum protection for the brain through its nutrients.

Multiple scientific studies have demonstrated that Mediterranean eating patterns lead to a 30–50% reduction in depression symptoms. The foods in this group contain minimal microplastic content while providing brain-protective omega-3 fatty acids along with antioxidants and additional health-promoting compounds.

The Road Ahead

The growing body of evidence about microplastics and mental health warrants immediate action. The proposed recommendations match established nutritional recommendations for physical and psychological health.

Researchers suggest creating a "Dietary Microplastic Index" that mirrors current dietary inflammation measurement tools to help people better manage their exposure levels. People should reduce their processed food intake, eliminate plastic from food preparation, and choose unprocessed whole foods until further research becomes available.

Your brain, along with your mental health, will express its gratitude through this choice.

Chapter 26: Beyond Stereotypes: The Exceptional Abilities That Make Autistic Minds Invaluable

According to The Lancet (in 2021), there were 61.8 million people on the autism spectrum in the world, which is equivalent to 1 out of every 127 people, amounting to a global distribution of 788.3 per 100,000 individuals.

Autism has been studied through the lens of deficits and challenges for an extended period. The world is designed for neurotypical minds, creating challenges for autistic individuals, yet their brains contain exceptional strengths that have produced numerous human innovations and discoveries.

Modern neuroscience research is transforming our understanding of autism by demonstrating that what were once considered limitations actually represent alternative, superior information processing methods. Our knowledge of autism has evolved from seeing it as a disorder to be fixed to recognizing it as a natural human neurodiverse variation that adds exceptional value to our communities. What are the areas where autism appears to hold an advantage over others without it?

Enhanced Pattern Recognition and Attention to Detail

Individuals with autism consistently demonstrate remarkable skills in detecting patterns and identifying details that often escape others. The autistic mind functions differently from typical brains when processing information, extending beyond basic numerical abilities. Research indicates autistic people excel at maintaining focus during extended periods while they identify intricate patterns in complex data, which neurotypical people tend to overlook.

The ability to focus on small details reaches beyond academic work. Autistic individuals demonstrate exceptional talent in quality control, software debugging, proofreading, and other fields that require precision. Their brains possess an innate ability to detect errors and inconsistencies that others typically overlook, thus making them essential for roles that require absolute precision.

As a medical consultant for Social Security Disability determinations, I worked alongside two men who appeared to be on the autism spectrum. They were superior in enabling consultants to ferret out inconsistencies in reports and ensure that they aligned with our agency's guidelines. One of them had an incredible, detailed knowledge of steam locomotives and the development of the national train system in the United States, and he visited railroad museums in his free time. In fact, he planned his free time around railroad exhibitions and conferences across the United States.

While attending a conference on sleep medicine, I was seated next to a woman who, spontaneously, told me that her husband, a highly reputable psychiatrist, was autistic. During this brief exchange, his attention was totally on the speaker, and he never turned once to interact with either of us. Yes, he was totally focused.

Systematic and Logical Thinking

Autistic minds demonstrate exceptional abilities in systematic thinking because they understand systems, analyze operational mechanisms, and identify governing rules across different domains. The cognitive style proves highly beneficial for fields such as engineering, computer science, mathematics, and scientific research. Autistic individuals solve problems through logical consistency, which differs from the intuitive and social cue-based methods used by neurotypical people.

The systematic method also applies to creative work. Autistic artists, alongside musicians and writers, employ structured methods to create complex and beautiful works through the exploration of methodical patterns, themes, and techniques.

Deep Focus and Specialized Knowledge

The development of intense, specialized interests, which scientists refer to as "special interests," stands as a significant strength. Individuals with autism who develop a strong interest in a subject tend to acquire knowledge that exceeds that of typical experts. The focused engagement of autistic individuals leads to innovative discoveries and new ideas. One outstanding example is Bill Gates, the pioneering computer expert who guided Microsoft to its success.

These deep interests, which some view as obsessive, form the foundation for outstanding scientific and technological achievements, as well as artistic and cultural contributions. The same trait that might be labeled "obsessive" during childhood will evolve into the powerful force behind pioneering research or artistic accomplishments in adulthood.

Honest Communication and Integrity

The direct and honest communication style of autistic people makes them highly valued by others. The autistic preference for direct communication stands out as refreshing and valuable in a society where social rules often hide the truth. Autistic individuals who maintain honesty and strong moral values become dependable colleagues and trustworthy team members.

Remarkable Individuals on the Autism Spectrum

Temple Grandin stands as the ultimate example of how autistic minds can create transformative change. During a time when autism understanding was minimal, Grandin received her diagnosis before becoming a global leader in livestock handling and animal welfare innovation. Through her visual thinking abilities, she gained the ability to see things from an animal's viewpoint, which resulted in innovations that decreased distress for millions of animals.

The curved chute system designed by Grandin for cattle handling has become a worldwide standard, while her insights about animal behavior transformed our approach to livestock management. Through her work, Grandin shows how autistic traits such as visual thinking and intense focus on animal behavior can produce innovations that benefit both animals and humans.

Satoshi Tajiri, who created Pokémon, revealed his autism diagnosis while explaining how his childhood insect collection hobby led to the development of a worldwide entertainment phenomenon. His systematic approach to understanding different species developed into a game concept that became popular worldwide.

Through his story, Tajiri demonstrates how special interests can develop into revolutionary innovations that change the world. His childhood obsession evolved into a business that now generates billions of dollars annually, bringing happiness to people from diverse cultures and age groups.

Greta Thunberg has revealed her autism diagnosis while explaining how her autism influences her environmental perspective. According to Thunberg, her autism provides her with exceptional climate crisis awareness because it eliminates social norms and unrealistic thinking. Through her straightforward communication style and dedicated focus on climate science, she has become one of the leading environmental activists today.

The social change initiatives of Thunberg prove that autistic traits, including focused attention, systematic thinking and direct communication, can lead to societal transformations. Through her ability to simplify complex information, she has started a worldwide movement that communicates essential truths.

Economist Vernon Smith, who received the Nobel Prize in Economic Sciences in 2002, has explained how his autism affects his research methods. Through his systematic thinking and attention to detail, he became a pioneer in experimental economics by developing laboratory tests for economic theories. His research introduced fundamental changes to how economists study markets, along with human behavior.

Academic fields undergo paradigm shifts through the contributions of autistic cognitive styles, as noted in Smith's work. Through his systematic testing of economic assumptions, he both challenged established beliefs and created new research possibilities.

Forward-thinking companies now understand the business value that neurodivergent employees bring to their organizations. The tech industry giants *Microsoft, SAP, and JP Morgan Chase* have established autism hiring programs because they understand that autistic employees bring competitive advantages to their organizations. These programs often involve tailored recruitment processes, inclusive environments, and ongoing support for neurodivergent employees.

In 2015, *Microsoft* established the *Autism Hiring Program* to recruit autistic people for full-time jobs. Candidates can also take advantage of their "*Interview Academy*" to get ready for their interviews. Established the *Google Cloud Autism Career Program* in 2021 with the goal of attracting and retaining autistic individuals within the cloud computing field. Working in tandem with Vocational Rehabilitation and PROVAIL, *HP's Spectrum Success Program* seeks out, interviews, and hires autistic individuals who meet specific criteria.

Beyond Individual Success: Collective Benefits

Autistic individuals contribute value to society that goes beyond their individual accomplishments. Their distinctive viewpoints generate solutions that benefit all people. Solutions developed by autistic individuals lead to user-friendly software and designs that accommodate sensory needs, thus creating more accessible products.

Research facilities now understand that autistic researchers bring valuable analytical abilities and precise attention to detail to their work. Autistic scientists across various fields, including astronomy and genetics, make discoveries that both expand human understanding and enhance life quality.

The recognition of autistic minds' exceptional abilities serves two purposes: it honors individual success while building a society that embraces neurodiversity. Educational systems need to adapt to different learning methods, while workplaces should provide communication accommodations.

Our growing understanding of autism beyond stereotypes will lead us to develop innovative solutions we have not yet conceived. The future will belong to diverse teams that unite different cognitive strengths and perspectives. The inclusion of autistic minds in our communities leads to both more inclusive environments and more innovative, successful, and creative communities.

Autistic individuals possess genuine strengths that enhance our world instead of being compensations for their challenges. Through neuroscience research and autistic voice listening, we discover that neurodiversity should be celebrated and utilized to benefit all people in society.

Chapter 27:
Young Boys, Societal Shifting, Violence, and New Mental Health Concerns

Significant global shifts in boys and young men are prompting serious conversations and heightened awareness of these mental health changes.

The world is waking up to significant cultural shifts that have had a profound impact on boys and young men growing up. Callous influencers are reportedly causing a crisis among young men, sparking debate on toxic masculinity and incels. Within this group of boys and men, crimes previously unthought of by young boys are increasingly making headlines worldwide, and society is asking, "Why?"

A recent Gallup poll, using aggregated data from 2023 and 2024, found that 25% of American men between the ages of 15 and 34 reported feeling very lonely the day before. This is far higher than the national average of 18% and the total for young women, which is likewise 18%. Is this sentiment related to what we are experiencing in the manosphere?

One question is, "What does the manosphere mean?" Are enough of us conversant to know what the term means and how it has impacted various aspects of our lives, including culture, law, and politics?

The word "manosphere" describes the vast network of anti-feminist websites, blogs, and forums that spread messages of male superiority and sexism. It promotes the unacceptability of emotions (see my article) and emphasizes power, wealth, and the inferiority of girls and women, who are considered mere tools for their pleasure.

The rise of the "manosphere" — a network of online communities promoting male supremacy and anti-feminist ideologies — has become one of the most pressing concerns for parents, educators, and policymakers in 2025. With the success of Netflix's drama "Adolescence" bringing these issues into mainstream discussion and ongoing concerns about misogynistic influencers like Andrew Tate, understanding how young boys are being targeted and radicalized online has never been more critical.

Understanding the Manosphere: Definition and Structure

The manosphere is an international network of social media influencers and communities promoting male supremacy and antifeminist ideologies. It encompasses various online groups that create, consume, and distribute content aimed at men and boys, all largely united by anti-feminist messaging. These communities discuss masculinity alongside topics such as health, gaming, politics, and finance but consistently frame their content through a lens that positions women and feminism as the root of men's problems.

What makes the manosphere particularly insidious is how it disguises hateful rhetoric through memes, comedy, and trolling, presenting extremist content as self-help, entertainment, and tools for financial success. This packaging makes it difficult for parents to identify harmful content and for children to recognize the extreme messages they're being exposed to.

The manosphere includes multiple interconnected groups with different focuses but shared anti-feminist philosophies. These range from "Men's Rights Activists" to more extreme communities like "incels" (involuntarily celibate), who view themselves as unsuccessful in obtaining romantic relationships and blame women for their perceived failures. Incels have become particularly notorious due to their association with real-world violence and their ideologies that view women as genetically inferior, manipulative and simultaneously owing men sex while being shamed for having sexual agency.

The Scale of Exposure Among Young Boys

Recent research exposes young boys to alarming levels of manosphere content. Hope Not Hate found that 80% of 16–17-year-old boys in the UK had consumed content created by Andrew Tate, the most prominent manosphere influencer. Even more concerning, 59% of boys accessed manosphere content through innocent and unrelated searches, meaning most adolescent boys will encounter this material without actively seeking it out.

The reach extends beyond individual influencers. Research indicates that 50% of young men aged 16–24 now believe feminism makes it more difficult for men to succeed, demonstrating how deeply these messages are penetrating young people's worldviews about gender relations and equality.

What I've found is that the manosphere is highly effective at targeting the legitimate fears and anxieties of boys and young men and then scapegoating women as the root of all their problems. This targeting is not accidental but represents a sophisticated understanding of adolescent male psychology and social media algorithms.

Video Games: The Gateway to the Manosphere

Video games play a particularly significant role in introducing young boys to manosphere ideologies. The connection isn't just about the games themselves but how gaming culture intersects with broader online ecosystems that normalize misogynistic attitudes.

Many video games rely on problematic gender representations that position "successful" men as strong, wealthy, aggressive, and heterosexual. Simultaneously, these representations depict women as highly sexualized objects or assign them to supportive roles. These stereotypical portrayals create a foundation where manosphere ideologies can take root and seem normal to impressionable young players.

Research on incels has shown how spending long periods on social media and gaming sites exposes young men and boys to incel content. Gaming becomes particularly dangerous when combined with social isolation. Too much time playing video games, along with a lack of a social life and limited interaction with women and girls, have been stated by men as reasons for identifying themselves as an incel.

The escapism that gaming provides can become a refuge where prejudice goes unchallenged, allowing harmful ideologies to flourish. Online gaming environments, which normalize misogynistic views and rarely confront them, provide comfort to many incels.

Social Media Algorithms: The Radicalization Machine

Social media platforms have become sophisticated tools for spreading manosphere content through their algorithmic systems. Due to platforms such as TikTok, X, and Instagram prioritizing engagement and profit over content quality or equality, algorithms further contribute to the spread of incel ideologies.

The mechanics of this spread are particularly insidious. Misogynistic content elicits intense reactions and controversial discussions, which tend to attract more likes, shares, comments, and views. Such content is therefore more likely to be recommended and circulated by algorithms, regardless of the harms it may cause. This creates a feedback loop where the most extreme and harmful content gets the widest distribution.

Social media platforms and search engines enable the manosphere's hatred of women and even profit from their content. Everyone has to be aware of the spread of this toxic misogyny and how it can radicalize young men and lead to real-life cases of harassment, violence, and mass murder.

The Podcast and Streaming Ecosystem

Podcasts have emerged as a particularly powerful medium for spreading manosphere ideologies. Video game streamers who espouse rightwing views often use streaming platforms like Rumble and social media websites such as X to spread gender-based hate. While some may not identify as incels or explicitly tell followers to join incel communities, their views align with incel ideologies.

The podcast format is especially effective because it can oversimplify complex social and political issues, risking misinformation and polarization. Unlike traditional media, podcasts often lack editorial oversight and can present extreme views as reasonable commentary. Some podcast personalities extend their influence by monetizing their personas, selling branded merchandise, offering premium content, and hosting subscriber-only events, creating financial incentives for increasingly extreme content.

These platforms regularly boast about being immune to "cancel culture." However, this means that they often allow streamers and influencers to disseminate misogynistic worldviews, conspiracy theories, and ideologies associated with the manosphere more broadly.

The Normalization Process and Psychological Impact

Repeated exposure across various platforms creates a strong normalizing effect. Men and boys' repeated exposure to social media that promotes incel ideology can normalize such perspectives. When young people encounter the same messages on gaming streams, TikTok videos, podcasts, and social media posts, these extreme views begin to appear mainstream and acceptable.

The manosphere employs an expansive lexicon designed to incite hatred toward women and fuel rivalry between men. Terms like "red pill," "alpha," "sigma," "beta," and derogatory language like "foid" (female humanoid) and "AWALT" (All Women Are Like That) create an insider language that reinforces group identity while dehumanizing women.

Much of the content spreading in the manosphere is based on disinformation or pseudoscientific theories that provide easy frameworks for men to assess their status while blaming women for their problems. For example, the "80/20 rule" refers to the pseudoscientific theory that 80% of women are only attracted to the top 20% of men, used to justify sexual and romantic rejection as women's fault rather than encouraging self-reflection or improvement.

The content also promotes dangerous physical transformations through "looksmaxxing" — extreme measures, including facial surgery, designed to increase perceived sexual value. These practices can lead to body dysmorphia, dangerous procedures, and unrealistic expectations about physical appearance and social success.

The manosphere creates multiple interconnected problems for society that extend far beyond individual attitudes and behaviors. Preliminary data suggest that the manosphere is encouraging sexist attitudes, exacerbating existing inequalities in schools, and spreading dangerous messages about mental health.

Violence and Extremism

There have been documented incidents of real-world violence linked to manosphere content. Groups within the manosphere, particularly incels, have been associated with multiple acts of extreme violence and even murder. While not everyone who engages with this content will commit violence, the ideologies actively glorify violence against women and normalize aggressive behavior as an essential part of masculinity. Picture the young men with the tiki torches in the Charlottesville incident.

The violence isn't limited to physical acts. Boys are repeating manosphere talking points in school and even harassing female teachers. The digital consumption of this content translates directly into real-world harassment and intimidation of women and girls.

Educational Disruption

Teachers report that gender equality has become one of the most challenging subjects to teach, with many students refusing to believe sexism is a real problem. The manosphere's influence has made classroom discussions about gender, equality, and respect increasingly challenging as students arrive with pre-formed hostile attitudes toward these concepts.

Mental Health Consequences

Paradoxically, while claiming to help men, manosphere content actually harms boys and young men by promoting unrealistic expectations, extreme physical transformations, and poor self-esteem. The content preys on vulnerabilities and insecurities of boys, especially those related to social isolation and sexual rejection. Still, it offers solutions that often worsen mental health problems and can lead to suicide in extreme cases.

The manosphere promotes a view of masculinity that is rigid, aggressive, and defined in opposition to women and femininity. This narrow definition of acceptable male behavior can be psychologically damaging for boys who don't fit these expectations or who have more complex emotional needs.

Evidence-Based Interventions and Solutions

Current research suggests several evidence-based approaches to help young boys and prevent further radicalization:

Parental Engagement Strategies

Parents need to actively engage with their children's online consumption. Research shows children are more likely to encounter harmful content when parents are less involved in their online activities. Specific strategies include:

Exploring Online Content Together: Watching content related to children's hobbies and sending them material you think they would enjoy can help train algorithms to promote more moderate content while also opening avenues for discussion. Engaging online with children should focus on understanding why they enjoy specific influencers rather than immediately intervening or critiquing.

Open-Ended Communication: Parents should ask simple questions, such as "How do boys in your class talk about girls?" or "Have you ever heard of...?" without judgment, thereby creating a safe space for discussion. What parents hear may be shocking, but approaching it with curiosity rather than dismissal helps maintain open communication channels.

Recognizing Warning Signs: Changes in how boys discuss women and girls, withdrawal from family and friends, and frequent use of manosphere terminology can indicate problematic influence. However, parents shouldn't panic if children use these terms occasionally, as they may not fully understand their meanings.

Media Literacy Education

Teaching children to be skeptical about online content can protect them from misinformation. This includes helping them question statistics, "academic" reports, and influencer claims they encounter. Research suggests that exposing children to misinformation with proper oversight can actually inoculate them against future manipulation.

Asking children why they trust specific influencers and where they think their friends get information helps develop fact-checking skills without seeming like formal instruction. The focus should be on developing critical thinking rather than simply prohibiting certain content.

Institutional Responses

Schools require more effective support and resources to address these issues. Recent guidance on teaching about misogyny in schools is welcome, but broader social institutions need to develop comprehensive interventions to prevent radicalization.

There's a need for more research on the specific mechanisms by which young people are influenced to join misogynistic spaces, including what specific streamers and influencers they engage with. Research on gender-based violence should explicitly inform government policy, addressing this as a gender-based issue rather than a general extremism problem.

Platform Accountability

Resistance or outright denial of their role in creating and maintaining this unhealthy culture of the manosphere is apparent. But, despite this obvious financial resistance, the research suggests urgent needs for digital platform reform:

Algorithm Reform: Platforms must prioritize safety over engagement in their recommendation systems, shifting away from algorithms that amplify controversial content solely because it generates interaction. In addition to the potential damage caused, the main issue is that profit motives are driving these platforms.

Content Moderation: All platforms should implement stronger policies against gender-based hate speech, ensuring consistent enforcement that does not use claims of protecting "free speech" as a way to evade responsibility.

Alternative Spaces: Creating positive online communities that offer belonging and male role models without toxicity, providing healthy alternatives to manosphere content.

Professional Support Systems

When concerning behaviors develop, resources are available, including mental health services through organizations like Young Minds, counter-extremism guidance, and government services like the ACT Early radicalization helpline. These services provide support without criminalizing young people, focusing on intervention and education rather than punishment.

The Path Forward

The increase in behavior associated with incel radicalization does not happen in isolation. Both offline and digital environments, including online games, which normalize misogyny and interconnected prejudice, lead to societies validating impressionable young boys' anger toward women.

Addressing this crisis requires coordinated action from multiple stakeholders. Parents need better tools and education to engage with their children's online lives. Schools require resources and training to address these issues in an age-appropriate manner. Digital platforms need to take responsibility for the content they amplify and profit from. Policymakers need to understand this as a serious threat to gender equality and public safety.

Most importantly, we need to provide young boys with positive models of masculinity that don't depend on the devaluation of women and girls. This means creating spaces where boys can explore their identities, process their emotions, and develop healthy relationships without being told that aggression, dominance, and misogyny are essential components of being male.

The research consistently shows that while the manosphere poses serious risks to young boys and society, early intervention, media literacy, and supportive family engagement can help protect vulnerable youth from its harmful influences. The challenge is to implement these solutions before more boys are radicalized and more harm is done to them and the women and girls in their communities.

Chapter 28: Understanding Sundowning: A Brief Guide for Families and Caregivers

The term "*sundowning syndrome*" describes a cluster of symptoms and behavioral abnormalities that manifest in a person's *altered state of mind, conduct, and mood* when the sun sets later in the day. It has been estimated that twenty percent or more of Alzheimer's patients experience sundowning at some point. To keep their care recipient comfortable and peaceful, caregivers must be aware of sundowning and have the necessary tools to manage it.

It's more of a symptom that people with dementia often experience than a disease itself. Estimates are that sundowning affects more than 60% of dementia patients, according to some research, while the actual prevalence varies greatly, ranging from 1.6% to 66% of dementia patients.

We may also be surprised by the current and future prevalence of the disorder. Someone develops dementia every three seconds, as noted by statistical tables related to the astonishing rate of population aging, and by 2050, there will be 152 million individuals living with the disorder.

Sundowning is a significant worry for families coping with dementia, and the wide variety of results illustrates that researchers have different ways of defining it. In other words, we have no accurate means of measuring worldwide sundowning or the many manifestations and behavioral symptoms that may be exhibited by individuals with it.

Changes in behavior that are often seen in individuals who are experiencing sundowning include:

Confusion

Paranoia and suspicion

Agitation

Frustration and anger

Hallucinations and delusions (auditory or visual)

Pacing or wandering

Restlessness

Anxiety or fear

A Neighbor of Mine

An elderly woman living with her husband in an apartment complex near me started experiencing sundowning. Although the man, who was in his mid-90s, remained fairly cognitively intact, the woman began to leave the building at night, as she said, "*I'm going to visit my parents."* She would often wander out without a coat, despite the cold night temperatures.

The woman was in her mid-80s and, after walking through the complex at night, would return to the building but be unable to enter because she didn't have a key. The husband had refused to give her a key in an attempt to keep her in the apartment, to no avail.

A woman resident of the building, noting the elderly woman's late-night exits, took it upon herself to shadow her to ensure her safety. Once she had returned to the building, the neighbor opened the lobby door for her, and she went back to her apartment. This went on for at least two months until a minister they knew decided to help find a safer place for them to live. They subsequently relocated to an assisted living facility, where they currently reside.

One theory proposed to explain sundowning behavior in Alzheimer's disease is the deterioration of neurons in a specific brain area that contains the body's principal circadian (sleep-wake) pacemaker.

Research has shown that sundowning exhibits different characteristics in different individuals. Among sundowning patients, agitation (56.4%), irritability (53.8%), and anxiety (46.2%) were the most common symptoms. The other manifestations can include confusion, restlessness, pacing, failure to follow instructions, suspiciousness, and hallucinations. The affected individuals either ask for more attention or withdraw and feel scared. These symptoms can also occur in the morning instead of the evening in some cases.

Who Is Affected?

Even though sundowning is most often associated with Alzheimer's disease and other dementias, it can occur in older adults who do not have dementia. People with sundowning disorder tend to be older, to develop dementia later in life, and to have more severe dementia and functional impairment.

The situation is very challenging for caregivers and families to handle. In fact, sundowning is the main reason why patients are placed in nursing facilities because of how difficult it can be to manage at home without the appropriate help and strategies.

Nursing homes have tried to meet this challenge by addressing sundowning and wandering in residents and usually require them to wear a special device around their wrist. The device activates an alarm system on the doors leading outside the building. For some, this may seem like an excessive means of control, but it is intended to prevent someone from wandering off, potentially with serious consequences.

I worked at a psychiatric hospital that did not have this type of system installed. One of the patients wandered off through an unlocked door and wasn't found until three days later. Unfortunately, this individual had become entangled in barbed wire near an adjacent farm, and the overnight freezing temperatures led to their death.

The Biology Behind Sundowning

Families who want to understand why sundowning occurs and which strategies might be effective should know how sundowning is related to biology. The human body has an internal clock system, which is approximately 24 hours long and controls sleep-wake cycles, hormone secretion, body temperature, and many other physiological functions. The brain contains molecular clockwork that governs these 24-hour rhythms (some sleep medicine specialists believe it's a 25-hour rhythm) and is reset daily by the light-dark cycle.

But the biological system that usually controls the body's functions in dementia becomes impaired. These processes involve genetic factors linked to specific genes, as well as neurodegenerative processes in brain regions that regulate the circadian rhythm. Research has now identified the brain pathways that connect tau protein pathology to sundowning-related disturbances, demonstrating how dementia affects brainstem neurons.

The Connection to Cognition

Sundowning is complexly related to cognitive function, and this relationship is multifaceted. The disorder is characterized by neurodegeneration, sleep disorders, disrupted circadian rhythms, and mood disorders. When the brain areas that regulate our internal clock degenerate, the body loses its ability to distinguish between night and day. The disruption affects more than just sleep patterns. The circadian system controls alertness, attention, memory consolidation, and emotional regulation, which are cognitive functions already impaired in dementia.

This desynchronization of the biological clock exacerbates existing cognitive problems, generating more confusion and stress. Typically, the brain starts preparing for sleep during the evening, which is probably why sundowning is at its worst during this time.

Healthy individuals experience a smooth and coordinated transition at this time. The impaired circadian system in people with dementia sends conflicting signals, which lead to the agitation and confusion seen in sundowning.

Strategies for Management

Although sundowning is challenging to handle, there are evidence-based strategies that can reduce its occurrence and intensity. The approach should be to work with the body's natural rhythms and to create a supportive environment.

The circadian system responds strongly to light, so providing appropriate lighting throughout the day can be beneficial. Bright light should be given during morning and daytime hours, and the lighting should be gradually dimmed as evening comes. Fluorescent lights at night should be avoided because they can be very disorienting.

The body's natural rhythms can also be reinforced by establishing predictable daily schedules. Meals, activities, and bedtime should occur at the same time every day. Simple evening routines that are calm can help the brain and the individual recognize that it's time to relax.

Daytime physical activities, especially in the morning or early afternoon, can help maintain a healthy sleep-wake cycle. Stimulating activities should be avoided in the hours leading up to bedtime.

Environmental Modifications

In the evening, create a calm, familiar environment. The volume and movement in the environment should be decreased, and the person may respond to soft music that they recognize. The temperature in the space should be suitable, neither too hot nor too cold, as temperature regulation can be affected in individuals with dementia.

The process of managing triggers requires identifying elements that tend to cause sundowning episodes. Fatigue, along with hunger, thirst, pain, and overstimulation, represents common factors that trigger sundowning episodes. Some episodes can be prevented through early management of fundamental needs.

Healthcare providers recommend that sundowning evaluations should be conducted regularly, and medical staff should employ a comprehensive approach to identify its risk factors. Caregivers need to collaborate with these providers to identify and address the causes of sundowning and evaluate treatment options, which may include personalized medications or behavioral interventions.

The Importance of Caregiver Support

Seeking assistance for sundowning management does not indicate failure, as it can be an overwhelming task for caregivers. The challenge can be best handled by receiving support through local groups, along with respite care and professional guidance that helps families facing this issue.

Keep in mind that sundowning is a brain-related symptom rather than a reflection of poor care quality or personal character flaws. Everyone involved in the care of someone who is sundowning needs to understand that they also need care. Burnout can be a serious consequence of attempting to handle this without assistance. That's where respite care for the caregivers comes into play.

I knew one woman who had a full-time day job while her mother, who suffered from increasing dementia, was at home alone. Other family members did not pitch in to help her, and she soon found herself having anger issues she had never experienced before. Burnout was evident.

I remember her telling me that she stopped herself from hitting her mother because of what the mother was doing in the home (a very distressing personal grooming issue). Calls to family members and support groups in the area ultimately resulted in the elderly woman attending a day program and being returned in the early evening. A family therapist was also assigned to the woman to help her cope with her mother.

Families can improve their approach to sundowning by understanding its biological origins in circadian rhythm disruption. Early identification of these sundowning patterns, combined with supportive interventions, leads to a better quality of life for individuals with dementia, as well as their family caregivers.

Chapter 29: Not Just Another Day in May 1970

American history is rich with tales untold and those too often told, but in a manner that is sometimes either unfaithful to the events or a sickening attempt to fatten the bottom line. Which was it when Urban Outfitters offered a replica of a blood-stained Kent State sweatshirt for sale at $130, a garment that is now being offered on eBay for $550? Is this a reminder of our recent, bloody past or someone's worse-than-crass attempt at "humor" in the service of corporate profit? Two words suffice: disgusting and shameful. **The corporation did pull the item from sale.**

Perhaps the designer was so poorly educated that he/she didn't fully appreciate what happened that May day in 1970 when four college students, exercising their right to assemble and protest, were gunned down by the local National Guard unit. Bleeding and dying on the college quad, one became the subject of an iconic photo that stands today as a symbol of presidential anarchy.

The president in question, Richard M. Nixon, a man who was almost disbarred for attempting to influence a juror when he was first admitted to the bar, deemed the students dirty hippies. Did hippies attend college? I thought they had "turned on, tuned in and dropped out," as Timothy Leary suggested was the appropriate reaction to political fascism in the form of Nixon.

I suppose you could say it was a "tribute" of sorts to those dead students, but I can't buy that. It was a distorted attempt at innovative design if you were not totally in touch with reality, I suppose. Similar to the recent shirt offered by yet another hip and edgy designer. The shirt, for those who missed it, was similar to the uniforms worn by the captives in the concentration camps in Europe during World War II. Oh, so trendy and creative, why would anyone protest? Lord knows except for the fact that more than six million people died while wearing those garments.

Gee, why not put out a Matthew Shepard t-shirt with, perhaps, a really gory, realistic portrayal of him being crucified on that Wyoming fence? Wouldn't that be too cool for words? Oh, yeah, they could sell it everywhere. Quick, what color scheme should we pick?

Or maybe a Harvey Milk shirt riddled with bullet holes? We could make a really nice jig with nails to simulate the bullets. Or was he shot in the head? If he were shot in the head, it would ruin the whole design. Must look that one up on Google. Thank God for Google; it lets us keep all that history stuff available, and we don't have to open even one book. Don't you love it?

Perhaps a clothing line called "Strange Fruit" with lots of really wonderful portrayals of African-American men hanging from trees? Wow, that would be great. You could position a few of them on one tree sort of like Christmas ornaments. Don't you just love it?

Maybe we might even go a bit more retro and dream up something with a civil rights theme? There's that wonderful trio (or was it four?) of little girls in the Birmingham church explosion, Mrs. Liuzzo, who was helping the Freedom Riders, or even Chaney, Goodman and Schwerner. So much to choose from during that era that you really had a hard time choosing.

Ask yourself who was sitting on their brains the day they decided that a Kent State sweatshirt was a good idea? How many people with an absence of good sense and decency were in the room when the mock-ups were passed around? Did not one voice speak out in protest?

The shirt is no longer being offered, but oh, how the melody lingers on for Urban Outfitters. How will you redeem yourselves, guys?

Chapter 30: A Reflex to Damage

Sports and all the training and repeated drills aimed at honing an individual's skills all depend on one thing: a reflex. No, this isn't the reflex you expect to see in a physician's office where they tap your knee or elbow with a rubber hammer. These reflexes are more dependent on your immediate, instinctual reactions that are almost unconscious. There are certain sports, however, where the reflex can become an impediment when not engaged in this actual physical and mental combat aimed at winning.

The success or failure in a sport is highly dependent on these reflexes. Some are intended to defend against a blow, others to quickly respond to a volley on a tennis court. Likewise, some sports are intended not only to develop a sense of self-confidence and personal mastery over emotional impulses but also a respect for others. There is no need in sports such as karate or aikido to be seen as more than the master of the execution of the moves as well as the master of one's self.

Asian martial arts are a personal physical and emotional journey of control over emotion with the knowledge that you could easily inflict a formidable injury, if not death, on any opponent. Killing, especially in karate, is ridiculously easy. This understanding of the danger in one's hands and feet is not to be taken lightly and must ever be under control. It's the same with prize fighters whose hands are considered lethal weapons.

Endless hours are spent in learning this control, and the masters constantly reinforce skill with restraint. The same is true in many other sports, of course, but in too many sports there is an emphasis on massive attacks on the opponent of the moment. The reflex is to injure, to stop at all costs, and to ensure the opponent will not be able to continue. Muscle is behind much of this effort as well as a credo to "rip their heads off," as I've heard high school coaches urge their football teams to do. It isn't a sport; it's a clash to demolish the opponent.

If you are constantly training to "rip their heads off" or you're paid a bonus for causing major physical damage to the other team, how do you put that philosophy into your pocket when you leave the field? The reflex you've been taught is always there, but you haven't received any of that special training found in the Asian martial arts, and that's where a major void exists.

Overriding all of this training are years of being pampered and "handled" when interpersonal problems arise off the field. There was always someone there to make sure you didn't fumble because you were a warhorse churning out billions of dollars every year for your owners. Yes, you have owners even though you think of yourself as having a contract. Lose the contract and you lose your livelihood, something you worked for your entire life. It isn't going to be pretty, but this sense of entitlement and the reflex were both there working against the sports workers.

New term, yes, but aren't they "workers," and aren't they chained to contracts that can be terminated for infractions (aka loopout for cancellation) or failure to produce? They are surely workers, just as anyone in an office is a worker. Call them athletes, if you must, but it's just another name for them. Yes, I dismiss all those years of toil to perfect their athletic skills, I know. Pare the skills away, if you can for a moment, and you have a worker. Just that simple, and without a job, what is a worker, especially one with no other skills than the one he used in the job he just lost? Unemployed.

The recent spate of domestic violence incidents among football players and even a judge in the South have, as the media is hammering home, opened a window into the private pain caused by this sense of privilege and reckless reflexes to damage. Perhaps there is good from bad again in the form of social media outcries to begin to take more stringent actions against the offenders and to help the objects of their viciousness.

The primary question now is whether there is true conviction or convenient public relations actions to quell the outcries. The game has changed, but we can expect that it may not change that much. Everyone has rights, and the athletes or others who fail to act in a civilized manner will sue whenever any action is taken against them. Major advertisers are already standing back, waiting to see just how strong and effective these new social media forces are or if they will die out given enough time and some tepid corrective actions.

The NFL had a mandatory course in domestic violence for new team members when Ray Rice joined the team. Now, it must be questioned as to the effectiveness of this program and how successful the new programs that are being formulated will be. It's not just domestic violence or violence toward others; a major change in personality seems to be needed. But how could any employer do this? Seems highly improbable, especially when the star athletes will still be pampered and protected for the good of the team and the corporate sponsors.

So where do they begin in order to address this particular psychological infection? It begins where everything begins, in childhood, but there's no going back for those adults who have lashed out in violence. They will have to look deeply into themselves and see who they are, if they can, and then take any actions they can to redress these egregious actions against women and children.

And let's help them with a beginning question for their inward look: What man beats a child to the point that he has a gash on his head and/or legs? And, for good measure, what type of man knocks a woman out and then drags her out of an elevator? Was she a match for him? Cheap shot in the extreme.

Chapter 31: Pedophiles Are the Nicest People

Take a moment to ask yourself a question. Do you know anyone who is a pedophile or a child pornographer? Give it some thought. Chances are, you may, but you'd never know it, just as the parents of six 10–11-year-old girls in a science class in an elementary school didn't know about their teacher. Highly thought of, respected, attentive to the students, you name it, this fellow had it in aces but it was all in the service of his predilection for sexually abusing young girls. We don't know if he also went after boys, but that's not the concern here. The concern is that pedophiles move among us easily and without a hint of suspicion. They are, in fact, those who are above suspicion.

The parents of a particular pediatrician in New Jersey never suspected that their wonderful, sensitive and oh-so-kid-friendly doc was also a pedophile until one mother filed a complaint after her daughter related an unpleasant touching incident in the exam room while she wasn't present. Later, his office computer was found to have thousands of child pornography photos on it, and, of course, he said he was "doing research," just as I've heard other pedophiles who used that explanation.

Of course, when your primary job is the supervision of young boys delivering the local newspaper, you have to wonder how qualified the guy I spoke to was in researching child pornography. In his home, however, he had at least three packed file cabinets with child pornography and then people began to question those overnight camping trips for the boys and the swimming lessons that involved diving off his shoulders.

Another case, where two young boys came forward to a relative about the fear and discomfort they had about their mother's boyfriend, was ultimately dismissed by the authorities. The reason? Simple. The kids had ADHD, and their stories couldn't possibly be believed even though they had, in private sessions, told more than one social worker and a child psychologist what had happened to each of them. The boys, by the way, never told each other what had happened to them. They were too ashamed and frightened that even worse things would happen to them.

The kids, for the time being, are living with a relative, but there is a remote possibility that they may be returned to the abuser's household. How do you handle that scenario without causing the children to "act out," as the school authorities like to say? But the courts, in their sometimes misguided wish to reunite families, do send children back into these familial torture chambers where they are physically abused and raped by men who have cleverly selected women with small children. Too many times, the children end up dead and the family is united at a funeral.

Do you know where one of the best places to find these vulnerable women might be for a pedophile on the hunt? Why, of course, it's Parents Without Partners. That is not to say that the groups don't actively try to protect group members from becoming prey for these monsters in sheep's clothing. But the true intent is so cleverly concealed that even these groups can be hoodwinked into providing entree to women with child victims. They also provide an unbelievable opportunity to rape vulnerable, single moms and they threaten to harm the children if the woman doesn't comply.

The American Academy of Child & Adolescent Psychiatry estimates that there are 80K reported instances of child sexual abuse each year, but this is far below the actual number. The reasons these crimes against children are not reported may be because the child fears the perpetrator, they have been warned that their siblings or parents will be harmed, the child is ashamed and is told they are to blame for the abuse, they fear retaliation by their parents or loss of love, and they are told no one will believe them.

Of course, there are too many instances of persons in the ministry who sexually abuse children, and they, for years, were protected by their orders, and no reports were made to the police. The trauma that ensues can result in many types of behavioral changes as well as depression and suicide. How should a person respond to any report of child sexual abuse? The Academy offers guidelines on their website.

Of one thing we can be sure: children are vulnerable. Trust is a wonderful thing, but children need to be helped to understand that not every adult is to be obeyed or to be trusted. That is not to say that children should be so frightened and intimidated that they respond with fear to everyone. It is not an easy task, but parents, guardians and persons in positions of authority need to help train children to be aware that they have rights and there are actions to be taken when someone does something that makes them uncomfortable.

When I was involved with one national organization, we talked to parents about "**Good Touch, Bad Touch**" and the need for a secret word to be used in emergency situations. The word was used whenever a stranger said a parent wanted them to go with them. "*What's the secret word?*" the child would ask. Then the child would immediately leave to seek safety in a neighbor's home, a store or a school.

Another was to train children to counter the popular ploy of a stranger asking a child to help them find their puppy. Kids don't immediately think about the peculiarity of an adult asking a child for help in finding a lost dog. Their response must not be a knee-jerk one of agreeing to help, and it takes training to ingrain this skill in the children's repertoire of responses. Just as you teach a child to read or to know their numbers, you need to teach them to act in situations of doubt.

Today, an ex-archbishop was arrested by the Vatican for sex crimes against children, and a science teacher in a New York City school was also arrested. Tomorrow it could be a police officer, a physician or a trusted neighbor, friend, coach, tutor or even a relative. Predators are everywhere, and they don't have easily distinguished signs that you can detect.

The moral is to let children know that they need to learn certain basic rules or actions for self-protection and for you to practice with them. Answer their questions with age-appropriate responses and always offer support and understanding.

Chapter 32:
Mammo Silence

The medical community continues to have a lively debate over the advisability of women over 40 having yearly mammograms. Women, meanwhile, seem to be left on the margins of the discussion, and for those with a strong family history of breast cancer, there is little wiggle room; they have to have one. Their concern is not whether they will develop breast cancer but when it might raise its ugly head, and they wait and wonder about their choices. For the time being, they sit quietly and opt for the mammo. A positive result turns the discussion to another contentious one: which procedure to have, be it a simple lumpectomy or a more radical surgery.

Now, it's not only having a mammogram but which one they should have. Yes, there are now regarding which test will most accurately aid them in their defenses against the monster. There is the regular mammogram, much like having your breast inserted into a waffle iron. No, it is not without some degree of discomfort. I'm not saying this to dissuade women from having one, but to make a point that I believe needs to be made.

The point here is, why is there any discomfort at all? Has technology not risen to the point where a graphic look into the tissue of a woman's breast can be obtained with no discomfort at all? Looking back to my college biology classes, I recall we could adjust our microscopes to look not only at the surface of a tissue on a slide but also into the middle and further back. All of it happened without ever flattening the slide sample.

The newer digital and now 3D mammo is, from a patient's viewpoint, just the same as the regular mammo: strip to the waist, insert breast onto plate, and have a second plate pressed hard to smash the breast. Some women complain of breast pain after either of these two. Other women say they've been bruised. I wonder how the female technicians feel about submitting women to this somewhat undignified procedure and the discomfort that it involves. The alternative, of course, taking a chance on breast cancer, is not an option most would want to consider. Make the appointment, go and give yourself a treat afterward for being health conscious.

The woman sitting with all the others who were lining the walls of the waiting room (all wearing not unattractive white robes with trapunto detailing on the sleeve edges and down the front) wondered aloud, "*Why can't they do it like they do in Italy? The doctor there just takes a small machine and runs it over the breast. No, nothing.*" She, of course, was referring to yet another technique, sonography. Sure, they can do that, but they often use both the regular waffle press and the slip of a unit over the breast.

Does one work better than the other? I don't think there's much discussion on the part of the women. They just accept that what must be done must be done, and that's it. Of course, in the course of submitting to the procedures, the women are also hoping against hope that everything will come out fine. It is the waiting for the reading and the report that is most painful.

The room was uncomfortably silent and unlike other waiting rooms at the hospital. Oh, yes, the 3D mammo is done at the hospital because the outpatient centers are finding it a bit too expensive right now, and they only have the digital mammo. No TV was on, no music was playing, and none of the women were seeking connection with others or asking questions or making comments about waiting. Nothing.

One woman stood out by her posture and positioning in her chair. Neatly coiffed, seated in her white robe, she rested her right hand, fingers outstretched, on her forehead as though deep in thought. Her face was a mask of controlled anxiety, and you couldn't help but wonder if she, unlike the others, had a feeling the exam results were not going to provide the relief she sought.

One nurse practitioner called the women, individually, after their procedures. Today she was working alone and would be doing this all day long for perhaps 40 women. There would be a simple list of questions regarding familial history of breast, colon or prostate cancer, then a breast exam, and that was it. Oh, did I forget to mention that part of this portion of the appointment was your signing a form that indicated you'd been instructed in the correct procedure for a breast exam? Well, you've had one today, and you could probably Google it if you chose to.

It's time to go, to give back your hospital tag, get a coin for the parking garage, and wait for 10 days for the written report. Until then, you wouldn't know how things had gone. A radiologist from an outside service, or one in Asia, would be reading your "films" and writing the report. You'll never see this person or know how qualified they are. You'll just get a report.

Chapter 33: No One Listens

Today, I was back up with my internet connection after a weekend of no service, and I was all set to post something on persons who feel helpless, but the actions of a certain physician on TV, the doc whose cameraman came down with Ebola, stopped me in my tracks.

After being, from what I understood, in "self-quarantine" in the interests of everyone here after her return to the US, the doc apparently felt she had had enough of that. According to one internet source (I haven't searched for ALL the resources), she was seen eating out. Ah, but she was in her car, not in a restaurant? Does that make it ok? Let me be clear here.

The first indication I had that she had left her home was when I saw that Whoopi Goldberg, on The View, blew up when she heard about it. Then I had to look into it. Rosie Perez also found it to be "irresponsible" of that doc, a former Big Pharma VP, to place the public at risk and to instill fear in the public. I very heartily agree. The doc isn't exempt from spreading the virus, and she had no way of really knowing much about this disease other than what she's read or been told. She's not a researcher as far as I know. Paid the big bucks may just have gone to her head this time, and it's now the business of the local police where she lives to bring her back into the barn.

Here's what the online article said: "*On Tuesday, NBC News President Deborah Turness said in a statement sent to staff members that (name of doc redacted by me) and her crew were doing well and in good health. While they are deemed to be at low risk, we have agreed with state and local health authorities that our team will not come to work, and they will stay at home taking their temperatures twice daily and staying in touch with the local health authorities for the remainder of the recommended 21-day period,*" Turness said.

(Name of doc) is not under any kind of mandatory quarantine order by the CDC or the state because she is at a very low risk of contracting Ebola. Any confinement is voluntary.

NBC did not respond to inquiries about the physician today, and the physician could not be reached for comment. You know, it's really comical, if you can see the black comedy here.

So, if Dr. So-and-So was acting so wonderfully in the interest of public safety, why did she need the dark glasses and hair pulled back? Disguise to protect her public image of sainthood? Did she really crave that take-out food so much, and is she so sure it was entirely prudent to do what she and her buddies did in the car in New Jersey? Nah, I don't think it was prudent at all, and, at the very least, it was incredibly BAD PR for her to do it. Now, she'll have the NBC talking heads put to the fire over this one.

Enough said about her. She'll have to explain this one until she's blue in the face, and we'll leave her to it.

Take stock of the things you've done already today. Did you get up this morning and fix yourself breakfast, take a shower, get your clothes ready, and then hop into the car or onto a bus or train? All pretty simple stuff, right?

But not for everyone. Next time you're in your home or your apartment, look around and think how easy it is for you to navigate these spaces, go up the stairs, easily glide through doorways, and get into your car. Even if you don't have a car, you have probably rented one, and it was all so simple and easy. You open the door, slide into the driver's seat, and off you go.

No need to have someone slip a transfer board between your wheelchair and the seat. No need to have your special hand clip adjusted so that you can push it onto the spinner on the steering wheel so you can drive. Oh, yes, of course, things are a bit different now, but for those who are paralyzed below the neck, they may breathe, but their hands aren't available to them as they are for us. Well, of course, they'll just have to get one of those nifty vans with the automated lifts that bring them right up in their chairs and put them into position. Easy as pie if you have what is it, $75K or more now?

Life is a series of "**challenges**," as we like to call them now. They aren't "**problems**" anymore because that's such a passé word, isn't it? Let's put a positive spin on things and see them as challenges to be met and conquered. Isn't that what all the news stories tell us? But what about the other "challenges" that are there but never recognized as such, or, if they are, they are somehow pushed back with slick words and tentative offers that never materialize in clear-cut action?

What am I thinking about? I went to a health fair today, and I sat at a table where the people were offering information to persons with disabilities. You know, those who have vision, sight or perhaps mobility problems. But for all the help that's there, it's the lack of follow-through that is most disheartening and frustrating.

Take, for example, the smallish woman in her early 80s who comes with two minor challenges. Her husband has Parkinson's, and he uses a walker. And they live in a small apartment complex where there are no cuts in the sidewalk for him to make the transition from their apartment to the small shopping center just a block away.

The frail couple must make their way another block or two in the opposite direction to the single sidewalk cut accessible to them. Then they have to walk in the roadway until they come across the next cut, which is now two more blocks away. Forget about the fact that the town is quickly gaining a reputation for pedestrian deaths and that, as a result, they have "secret" pedestrians trying to ticket people who don't stop for pedestrians in the roadway.

The roadway is more than dangerous. It is an invitation to hospitalization, except for the fleet of foot. The couple take their physical health and their very lives in their hands each time they attempt a simple trip to the deli nearby. But it doesn't stop there. Yes, of course, they've spoken to the mayor, the man in charge of public works (the state gave funds for sidewalk cuts), and the owner of their apartment complex. The unanimous response from all of those empowered to help them? There are other priorities, but they'll get around to it.

Or, they've heard nothing at all. They've been ungraciously ignored as unimportant, and their lives have been seen as expendable. Who cares if another elderly couple disappears into the recesses of some hospital or nursing home? The rent can go up, and younger people can move in who won't ask for sidewalk cuts. Another challenge solved.

The woman had another request. Could someone tell the buildings department that the iron stanchions around the entrance to the supermarket wouldn't permit entrance with a walker? *"Even if they would only take one of them out,"* she pleaded, *"it would make it easier for my husband and anyone with a carriage or wheelchair."* But, as she continued, *"Everyone complains, but I'm the only one who says anything about it."* They don't listen, and the grumbling continues with the continuing inaction or lack of voicing to those in authority. She speaks not just for herself and her husband. She speaks for all of them.

Try using a walker for a day and see how you do. And remember those sidewalk cuts when you do. Lack of such cuts and lack of a sidewalk leading into the parking lot of a major supermarket chain resulted in a woman in a motorized wheelchair being hit by a car as she navigated the slanted driveway into the parking lot. Why was she in the parking lot? Ah, you see, it's the only way you can get to the front entrance of the store. There is no other way. It's surrounded by a parking lot. In case you're interested, the woman suffered two broken legs and other injuries. The supermarket still hasn't installed a sidewalk, cuts or no cuts.

Is there anything else? "*Yes, they told us that we have to get an internet phone because they're removing all, what is it, the copper wire and we won't have a phone if we don't switch.*" Challenge there? "*Yes, we don't have cable because we can't afford it, and with my eyesight, it's useless.*"

What she didn't know, of course, is that when the electricity goes out, so does the cable, and along with it any cable phone services. This, then, leaves her and everyone else with an internet or cable phone without any way of getting help in this time of emergency. This frightening scenario was played out during Superstorm Sandy in 2012 when some areas were without electricity for two weeks or more.

How many people in their early 80s or their 90s are now being frightened into buying a service that they don't need? The phone is their lifeline to family, friends and vital services. They couldn't live without it. That is what the cable customer service representatives are counting on: fear. It is a potent sales technique when used correctly.

Who else is going to try to fleece our seniors for their own corporate convenience and stockholders' wishes? The elderly are getting it from all sides, and when they have a disability, as most of them will, it's worse.

Everyone has a cell phone, correct? No, because enough of the elderly can't afford that, too. Want a phone with larger letters and really adjustable volume for those with increasing hearing loss? That will set them back $200 at least. Want one that also has a screen where they can read large type if they can't hear the conversation? Don't ask what that will cost. And isn't it wonderful that the phone service only costs $160 a month? Oh, my, that is a real dent in their monthly Social Security check.

The world of the elderly is shrinking even as we see this group expanding in size. Services are popping up all over the place, but who will pay for them? Do people really have such unrealistic ideas about the financial situation of elderly persons? I think they do. And, when it's all said and done, how can we hold our heads up and allow this to happen to the Greatest Generation?

Chapter 34: Transport Yourself Into Your Family's Future

Photo albums were the stuff of family memories with yellowed and often torn photos of people without names. Standing stiffly on prop sets intended to provide a bucolic view for the folks back home in Europe, we marveled at their clothes, the mustaches and their erectness. Of course, in many instances they had to stand erect because the huge cameras demanded a rigid pose while the glass plate was exposed to capture the image.

Photography advanced; we bought new cameras, and family fun was now the stuff of our albums, which still had the photos carefully imprisoned in little white tabs at each corner. Still, unless someone remembered to place a name and a date in white ink on the black matte surface, our only recourse was to find a family friend or relative who knew who these people were. After awhile, this becomes much more difficult as people move away, forget or die. Then we are left with books of photos of unknowns who may or may not be related to us.

More advances and a bit more income meant families bought rudimentary movie cameras and then moved on to more sophisticated equipment as the science progressed. We are now in an era where choosing the right format might mean the difference between reviewing those old photos and videos or not having access at all.

I have heard that the Library of Congress has taken on the enormous task of keeping one of every type of input device in its inventory so that they will always be able to read what they are storing. So, goodbye stereopticons, Zip Disks, A drives, microfilm, microfiche, big and little floppies, and CD/DVDs, and hello USBs and external HDs. What's the next media coming down the road? Whatever it is, we have to be ready to convert, convert, convert to ensure we will be able to recover.

Now comes the interesting part where all this techno tedium gets to give us the golden memories. What good is technology if you aren't being creative in your memory-making activities? Okay, the latest idea (and I think it's a honey of an idea) is the "ethical will." Nah, I don't like that "will" idea so much, and I don't even think you need to use the word "ethical." What are you, some kind of memory ripoff artist trying to skew those golden moments in the service of what?

Work on collecting family memories from the people involved in them right now or in the not-too-distant past. Sit them down or take your cell, videocam or DSLR, write out a short series of questions regarding family history, and you're on your way. And you shouldn't concentrate exclusively on the older members of the clan. Get the younger members into the whole scheme, and doing a year-by-year family docu might be really interesting. Length is up to you, but I wouldn't be too quick to edit things down because it removes that element of reality that you want. You are looking for the real, not the slick. Pull out mementos and let people mull over them.

The current range of software to produce this opus is vast, and you needn't saddle yourself with Final Cut Pro or Premiere Pro, either. Take a look at something that has a short learning curve, can do quick and easy editing, and can even add a voice-over or music. It can be done simply, and it doesn't take experience. Do a Google search.

Begin your family history now and let everyone in on the project. It's fun, it's educational, and it's for the future members of your family, so give them something they will truly treasure. It's the gift of you.

Chapter 35: The New College Grind Isn't the Classes

College, in the minds of those who may have been fortunate enough to graduate 20–30 years ago when the American dream was in full flower, is a time of facts, fun and nose-to-the-grindstone courses and exams. It was pledging for sororities or fraternities, going to dances, Spring break and first loves. All of it is such a bit of gossamer fluff that it might have been the stuff of a Hollywood movie or one of those "let's put on a play in the barn" types that made household names of teen stars. It ain't so today if it ever was then.

Nostalgia must come to terms with what our current crop of college students face and the picture isn't a very pleasant or bucolic one. Today, I came face to face with one of those realities of which I had been ignorant because I was always an evening student, one of those odd birds with one foot in a full-time day job and evenings spent as a college student. I didn't go away to school, never lived in a dorm (except when I taught graduate students during several summers) and had no idea about food plans. I ate at home, made my own meals and, like so many, took out a few loans to get by.

While waiting to have my hair cut today, I passed some time with an older patron as we began first talking about the ravages of Super Storm Sandy and the grief it brought into the lives of so many families, the cost of flood insurance and the new requirements for any home in the redrawn flood plane. Then the subject turned to college and her godchild who was told, now that she had completed her sophomore year, that she had to move out of the dorm, find her own apartment and was no longer eligible for the meal plan. "She's a good kid who works at Starbucks and does the best she can. Her parents don't have the money to pay for school."

I had never heard about this Remove Yourself From the Dorms rule and the woman told me that, yes, it was something that many colleges did. "Don't they want her to finish college," she asked. It was going to be even more difficult now that she would have to find at least three roommates, pay more money for meals and still work while trying to pay her increased rent in addition to other incidentals. This young woman had been barely scraping by and now they were making it harder. What could be the reason. I couldn't think of one. Was this the college administration's version of "tough love" or something?

It sounded like something seemingly benevolent dads did when they wanted to teach their kids to swim; they threw them out of the boat. It was sink or swim time for this young woman and I wondered what it would do. Her grandparents had offered her a room in their home, but it wasn't in the state where her college was. She'd have to transfer, but then she'd have to pay out-of-state tuition for at least two years and, if all went well, that would be just when she would be graduating, if she would be graduating.

Recent grads are swimming in a tsunami of student loan debt that will hit this country as it crests ever higher and students can no longer pay because they cannot find jobs that will enable them to pay OR they can't find jobs at all. College was supposed to be the way to "make something of yourself." The illusion appears to be becoming yet more unpalatable as college tuition goes up and job prospects go down. Why take out loans for a life of unpayable debt and an ineligibility to gain relief through bankruptcy? What's more, why even go to college if technical skills and not an education are what the marketplace wants from young workers?

I gave it some thought and then I recalled a similar conversation I had about college with someone in the media. His children had graduated from Ivy League colleges and now one son was headed, upon graduation, to a job on Wall Street and would be sharing a million-dollar condo with a few friends. How different the circumstances were between this young woman and that man's son. Could she have contributed to a Wall Street firm's corporate earnings or world advancement? Perhaps, but she would never get the chance because she didn't have the parents who were wealthy graduates of prestigious colleges and family friends in places where she could benefit from these connections. It was more than unfair but she needn't know about this scenario. She had enough to juggle right now just trying to get her degree.

Oh, and did I forget to mention that she's been on the dean's list every single term and that she chose to go to a brick-and-mortar school where she'd have real interactions with her professors? She isn't going to take a degree from a diploma mill, buy her term papers (even if she had the money) or try to pass herself off as something she's not.

But there are those who will and they'll get jobs where they lie on their resumes (some in the most outrageous fashions) and become well-heeled consultants. And, yes, I did hear of one spectacularly successful person who engaged in all of these unseemly activities and managed to cage top positions on college boards and corporations. Amazing what a little chutzpah and no background checks will do for a larcenous career.

Let's hope she never finds out the truth about any of this because she's been disappointed enough by the whole college experience.

Chapter 36: The Art of the Hidden Message

A ladybug keeps trying to set up a cozy spot for the cold winter nights ahead, and this little creature has decided that my living space is the exact perfect place for it to be. I've tried at least three times to carefully scoop it up with a paper towel, making a little basket to catch it as I inch the paper along the wall beneath it and then bringing a bit of the top over it until it falls into the scoop. It's delicate work because, while I want the little bug out, I don't want to harm it. Out the window I toss it, but it keeps coming back. Such determination, or maybe it's just opportunity that it sees.

All of this might be a metaphor for things that go on around us every day, and it really hit home tonight as I, in my determination not to get caught up in election returns, watched a few "House of Cards" episodes. It's incredible how my efforts toward the ladybug and the congressman's actions on the Hill are so similar. We both want our way. I don't want harm, and maybe he doesn't either, but he's capable of it when he deems it necessary.

The mix of politically themed TV shows should more appropriately be called a rash of shows with the same theme. It's the "Bonanza" of this season, but there are more wily people here than you would find on the Ponderosa in a decade. Straight shooters have gone the way of pull chains in bathroom plumbing, and the new batch of characters has to spend endless nights trying to outfox each other. Just following the machinations can be taxing, but it's also a veritable chess game that draws you in as you watch the moves that are or are not anticipated. The end game is, of course, taking over the board with your perspicacity.

I can't help but wonder how much of the plots border on what the writers have heard or been fed by people in the know in Washington, DC. Is there really a cleanup woman who is so totally adept in any messy situation that she knows exactly what to do to get the desired result? That, of course, would be "Scandal." I have seen at least two episodes and haven't become a fan. Maybe I just can't swallow that suspension of disbelief that is so necessary to liking these shows.

Watching "Breaking Bad," I became a critic of too many "fade to black" scene changes and then an extraordinary action that was never explained. For example, how did Walter White get that ricin into the sugar substitute packet so that he could kill that woman? The man is a genius magician besides being more than a top-notch chemist/meth cook.

I saw a bit of "Madam Secretary," but that didn't catch me, either. Yes, the clothes fit so well, and everyone is so smooth that it's irritating, and they live in such great places. Sure, that's what it's really like, isn't it? After all, Mitch McConnell did live at the Ritz-Carlton in Washington, DC and those are some pretty nice digs. I've stayed there on at least one occasion and on another at their hotel in Laguna Niguel, California. Luxurious. What a background for skullduggery.

What I think just might be the value in these shows is that they provide us with a great understanding of just how to be really successful at being underhanded. I'm sure that comes in real handy in business these days and even in education, where you might want to wheedle your way into a cushy administration slot. But then, this was all anticipated years ago with "The Peter Principle," where even the truly mediocre rise to the top by virtue of just staying put. I have seen examples of this. But I've also seen the unbelievably ruthless get to positions of power by cutting everyone else off at the knees, so to speak. They do it so cleverly that the victims never see it coming, or, if they do, they know they are powerless to do anything to stop it. The groundwork has been carefully laid, as it always is by Congressman Frank Underwood in Cards.

We can see the shows as entertainment, or we can see them as training. Those looking for seminars on how to bring Sun Tzu into business will find them instructive as well as entertaining. So, you don't have to read and reread "The Prince" or "The Art of War" in order to learn guile. Just watch TV and be sure to absorb all the hidden messages.

I wonder if the ladybug will be back tomorrow.

Chapter 37: One Shining Light Is Out: Mike Nichols

Mike Nichols' death was reported today, and I'm sure that throughout the entertainment field or anywhere someone enjoys creativity and invention and entertainment for adults, it resonated deeply. He was one of the premier talents of his time, and his works will inspire and cause us to think as well as to laugh for millennia to come. Mike Nichols now belongs to the ages, and I, for one, am very glad I had an opportunity to see his work early on when he first began performing with the very talented Elaine May at New York's Golden Theatre.

Nichols and May provided my extremely wonderful entrance into becoming a regular New York City theatergoer, even if I sat almost against the wall in the balcony. It was a magical event in my mind. I didn't know how to dress, what would be expected of me and how or whether I'd fit in.

Yes, I grew up in the wilds of Queens, and we didn't have theater there even though my town had five movie theaters. A version of summer stock would come after the vaudevillians had left and were forgotten. But we still had remnants of vaudeville when I was much younger, and I'd seen many. When you went to the movies on Saturday morning, in addition to 10 cartoon features and a double feature film, you had to sit through god only knows how many vaudeville acts. Doesn't that sound ancient now? It sure does to me.

Broadway was a place we all knew existed, but none of us had ever been there. You only went anywhere near Broadway when you got a job in Manhattan, and then you discovered two-fers that meant cut-rate tickets to shows. I don't think Nichols and May were two-ferred, but I got the tickets, I am forever grateful.

As soon as the couple came onto the empty stage the magic began and it continued without a break until they suddenly turned the tables. Looking out at the audience, Mike asked for ideas for an impromptu skit they would create right there without preparation. The suggestions came fast and loose, and he gleaned several immediately. They'd pick a situation that was posed, improvise the skit without any discussion, and go on to the next without missing that proverbial beat. It was marvelous! I was in love with the theater, and I've never lost that love.

When they broke up, I was mystified because they were so perfect together and they played off each other so effortlessly. But each went their way. It was a moment in time, and then it was gone, but oh, what a moment. Some things, I guess, live out their lives, and then it's on to something else.

Nichols would go on to amaze us with the breadth of his talent in film and TV. Sure, he'd have misses, but when he was on his game, as he had been that night in the Golden, he was unbeatable. I do have the LP album of the performance, and I treasure it even if I currently do not have a turntable and ancillary equipment to do it justice. The album stands as a rare piece of entertainment Americana that I treasure. That night was my theatrical christening, and we do try to keep something from these momentous occasions, don't we?

RIP Mike Nichols I'm sure glad I got to have the experience you provided.

Chapter 38:
Cosby: Another
Icon Crumbling?

Icons enjoy incredible trust from us, and we defend them, sometimes savagely, when there is an attempt to knock them off their revered pedestals. But what happens when this trust may be incredibly abused and in no way deserved? Do we shut our eyes to the facts, or do we take one of two tracks: defend them against all odds or look at any compelling evidence? It really depends on what motivates you to hold them in high regard in the first place, doesn't it? This is an intensely emotional issue where fact and fantasy spar with our minds, and the devil is often in the details—to which we may still remain blind.

Bill Cosby was always a wonderful image for all of us and I enjoyed his humor, his TV shows and his stand-ups. I liked him in "I Spy," and whatever he desired to do, even those pudding commercials. He was a man of dignity, character and an inspiration to all of us. We wanted a dad like him, a physician like him, and a genuine, understanding friend like him. If what we are hearing from a string of women is true, we have been misled, and even some of the media are admitting they, too, may have played a part in this charade. Yes, of course, it's still in the conjecture stage, and definitely no depositions will be taking place on the advice of attorneys and PR people. Depositions are where those devils lie in wait.

Color didn't play into the issue for me. Didn't matter. I even got intense enjoyment out of "Que Pasa, USA," a Spanish-language TV show with a wonderful family. And no, I don't speak Spanish, but I could follow the family and enjoy the show just the same. Steven Bauer was a great foil in this loving family. He, of course, has gone on to "Breaking Bad" and "Ray Donovan."

What is playing out in Cosby's case, as we've seen it in many others, is that "he said," "she said," but, of course, after viewing the NPR video, he's not saying because "we don't talk about that." Camille sat by him smiling as though he were discussing another pudding commercial he had planned. We've seen the dutiful wife stand by other men. I don't have to count the ways beginning with Bill Clinton and Paula Jones, Jennifer Flowers and then Monica Lewinsky. He even sat with Hillary on a couch, prior to his election, and denied any affairs in a now-famous TV interview.

Infidelity doesn't play very well with voters or family-oriented entertainment features on TV. So, when something like the Cosby dustup happens, it sends ripples through homes across the nation and causes network executives to rethink their program plans. Apparently, that has happened.

But why are we so upset? We know that many politicians we've revered were serial adulterers, and yet we retain an incredible admiration for them. President Kennedy leads the pack, although he wasn't alone in his serial affairs. He and the others had a cooperative press shielding them from our scrutiny. A bit of digging on your part will turn up some surprises about presidents and others.

The difference with Cosby isn't so much that he's a family-oriented, pop-of-the-nation entertainer; it's the backstory that his appetite included something we only find in people like Max Factor cosmetics heir Andrew Luster. Cosby's allegations aren't about infidelity per se, but drugging and raping women. It's the drugging part that we find most abhorrent, if true. Rape is bad enough, but when the active drugging of a woman or a man is involved, it reveals something, I believe, that is sinister about the person in question. Certainly, Luster is the poster boy for this type of egregious behavior, and he may spend 125 years in jail for his actions.

What do we take away from all of this? People are human with good and bad qualities, and some, if not many, marriages arrive at certain understandings about individual behavior. We know there are marriages of convenience or ones that are purely to create a certain image or advance a career or gain social prominence. Some are created to promote a political agenda. Royals have been doing this for centuries.

We have no right to judge them because we aren't involved. It's their lives and they are entitled to live it however they wish but, when it comes to criminality, I think we have a different view of the person. Certainly, when someone presents themselves as a pillar of family morality and preaches to others about how they should live their lives, we find this repugnant if the allegations are true. Will we ever know? Who knows?

Chapter 39: Psychologists Guided Torture for CIA

P sychologists have a code of ethics that clearly states what we may not do in our professional lives and yet, for some, these are merely words just as the Hippocratic Oath is merely meaningless verbiage for some physicians. The guiding principle for those who clearly veer off the designated path of ethical behavior is, of course, that ever-famous motto of "Show me the money!" I suppose it is true that everyone has their price, but I still cling to the belief that it's not true. Some of us still believe in the moral imperative not to do evil. We don't need to hark back to the Germany of the 30s because we have perversity working full tilt right here in the good old USA.

Although only two psychologists have been singled out as the ultimate culprits and thought-leaders in the horrendous torture campaign run by the CIA, there is, by some accounts, at least five or so others who worked in the same company. I cannot believe that they weren't, in some measure, also involved and aided in the ultimate presentation provided to an incredibly gullible CIA purchasing agent.

Ever since we first learned of the existence of this ultra-secret agency (thanks to a fool with a gun), intelligent readers have come to view it as the counterpart of "anything goes" in "protecting" this country. Yes, anything seems to have been permitted despite the objections of those who understood interrogation techniques and had a knowledge of who they were interrogating, Al-Qaeda operatives.

The behavior of James Elmer Mitchell and Bruce Jessen (both nicely ensconced in mega-mansions on either Coast of the USA) is cogently laid out in an article written by Michael Daily in The Daily Beast. Read it and get your fill of this vile, totally unacceptable behavior by men who were supposed to help people, not hurt them. Curious how this happened.

Let me put a bit of perspective from the point of some psychological research into it. It doesn't condone it, but it tells you where the seeds were planted and then transformed into a program for torture. Think of it as though it were pediatricians who deliberately deformed babies just to see that they could do it and then got paid a king's ransom to do it. Ugly, I know, but it's the closest I can come to this brutality and shameful behavior.

Mitchell sat at the knee of famed psychologist Dr. Martin E. P. Seligman who, while at The University of PA, ran a series of experiments with puppies that was aimed at working out the theory of depression development. Actually, he wasn't interested in puppies, but in college students who were experiencing depression and he wanted to devise a way to help them.

The result of Seligman's work was that early experiences of either being helpless in a situation or of learning to survive these experiences led to depression or a resistance to depression. We couldn't go back and change early childhood experiences, but we could help people change their behavior through the technique now known as Cognitive Behavioral Therapy (CBT).

The theory of learned helplessness and Mitchell's craven praising of Seligman led to more discussion and the result was Mitchell's corruption of the original work into a means of incredibly inhumane torture. Not only would he plan a program, according to some reports, he would gladly supervise it. What soulless individual does something like that? I can only compare it to what was done by Dr. Josef Mengele in Nazi Germany where he injected dye into the eyes of Jewish prisoners to see if he could change them from brown to blue. Medical experiments? No, brutish, incredibly disgusting corruption of his medical training.

What must other psychologist researchers be thinking about this torture program and the psychologists who participated and what of The American Psychological Association's reaction? My mind goes back to two works, one well-known, the other not so. The not-so-well-known work by Max de Crinis resulted in the Euthanasia Decree signed by Hitler to rid the world of "undesirables."

The second, very well-known experiment performed at Stanford University, was The Stanford Prison Experiment where the experimenter, Dr. Philip Zimbardo, a social psychologist, became so wrapped up in his study that he lost his professional perspective. He actually believed, for a short time, during the experiment that he had to prevent students from "escaping" from the experimenter-constructed jail at the school.

Forget that at least one student had a psychotic break, others had medical consequences and who knows what else. Zimbardo claimed he adequately debriefed everyone at the end of the experiment and went dancing off into the sunshine of his professorship. OK, Phil, but what about the neighbors who were also involved in seeing students handcuffed at their homes and pushed into police cars or the long-term consequences of PTSD which, I'm sure, there were? How has that played out for you? Still have an absolutely guilt-free conscience about all of this? I won't go into your experiment into hypnosis which was described in a Sunday NYT magazine article years ago.

While we're at it, consider the Dr. Stanley Milgram "Obedience to Authority" experiment at Yale. He subjected naive people (call them experimental subjects) to thinking they'd killed someone with an electric shock. Women's results were tossed from the experiments because Milgram felt they provided results that weren't in line with his thinking. Oh, yes, all of this was done to see whether ordinary people could be induced to kill someone a la the Nazis during WWII. The work came directly out of that era. Milgram debriefed the subjects later and showed them they hadn't killed anyone, but what of the woman who shouted at her husband that he was no better than Eichmann? Remember Adolph Eichman who signed the travel orders to send Jews to the gas chambers?

What a wonderful legacy psychology has. I thought we'd learned but there appears to have been inadequate attention paid to psychologists' mistakes and their casual dismissal of questionable experiments. No, I didn't mention the experiment where students were actually injected with adrenaline.

I've heard of some pretty egregious behavior on the part of psychologists and psychiatrists, but the current CIA report indicates we've hit a new low with incredible rewards for the perpetrators of this tawdriness. None of the questionable work that preceded it justifies this in any way, nor am I trying to offer anything other than examples of how psychologists failed those who came to them to help in research.

I remember being in a graduate program where we were required to volunteer (not really the right word, but they used it anyway) for 10 hours of experiments in order to pass our course. There was a large board listing all of the requirements to get into each experiment and also what would disqualify you. I looked for everything that said "no paid" and allowed people wearing glasses. I did my 10 hours in boring memory experiments run by doctoral students and I know they must have wanted to pull their hair out. I was not a willing subject and they knew it.

So, how do you get honest responses from people who are being forced, coerced or tortured (as in the case of the CIA)? You don't.

Chapter 40: Psychologists Guided Torture for CIA

Psychologists have a code of ethics that clearly states what we may not do in our professional lives and yet, for some, these are merely words just as the Hippocratic Oath is merely meaningless verbiage for some physicians. The guiding principle for those who clearly veer off the designated path of ethical behavior is, of course, that ever-famous motto of "Show me the money!" I suppose it is true that everyone has their price, but I still cling to the belief that it's not true. Some of us still believe in the moral imperative not to do evil. We don't need to hark back to the Germany of the 30s because we have perversity working full tilt right here in the good old USA.

Although only two psychologists have been singled out as the ultimate culprits and thought-leaders in the horrendous torture campaign run by the CIA, there is, by some accounts, at least five or so others who worked in the same company. I cannot believe that they weren't, in some measure, also involved and aided in the ultimate presentation provided to an incredibly gullible CIA purchasing agent.

Ever since we first learned of the existence of this ultra-secret agency (thanks to a fool with a gun), intelligent readers have come to view it as the counterpart of "anything goes" in "protecting" this country. Yes, anything seems to have been permitted despite the objections of those who understood interrogation techniques and had a knowledge of who they were interrogating, Al-Qaeda operatives.

The behavior of James Elmer Mitchell and Bruce Jessen (both nicely ensconced in mega-mansions on either Coast of the USA) is cogently laid out in an article written by Michael Daily in The Daily Beast. Read it and get your fill of this vile, totally unacceptable behavior by men who were supposed to help people, not hurt them. Curious how this happened.

Let me put a bit of perspective from the point of some psychological research into it. It doesn't condone it, but it tells you where the seeds were planted and then transformed into a program for torture. Think of it as though it were pediatricians who deliberately deformed babies just to see that they could do it and then got paid a king's ransom to do it. Ugly, I know, but it's the closest I can come to this brutality and shameful behavior.

Mitchell sat at the knee of famed psychologist Dr. Martin E. P. Seligman who, while at The University of PA, ran a series of experiments with puppies that was aimed at working out the theory of depression development. Actually, he wasn't interested in puppies, but in college students who were experiencing depression and he wanted to devise a way to help them.

The result of Seligman's work was that early experiences of either being helpless in a situation or of learning to survive these experiences led to depression or a resistance to depression. We couldn't go back and change early childhood experiences, but we could help people change their behavior through the technique now known as Cognitive Behavioral Therapy (CBT).

The theory of learned helplessness and Mitchell's craven praising of Seligman led to more discussion and the result was Mitchell's corruption of the original work into a means of incredibly inhumane torture. Not only would he plan a program, according to some reports, he would gladly supervise it. What soulless individual does something like that? I can only compare it to what was done by Dr. Josef Mengele in Nazi Germany where he injected dye into the eyes of Jewish prisoners to see if he could change them from brown to blue. Medical experiments? No, brutish, incredibly disgusting corruption of his medical training.

What must other psychologist researchers be thinking about this torture program and the psychologists who participated and what of The American Psychological Association's reaction? My mind goes back to two works, one well-known, the other not so. The not-so-well-known work by Max de Crinis resulted in the Euthanasia Decree signed by Hitler to rid the world of "undesirables."

The second, very well-known experiment performed at Stanford University, was The Stanford Prison Experiment where the experimenter, Dr. Philip Zimbardo, a social psychologist, became so wrapped up in his study that he lost his professional perspective. He actually believed, for a short time, during the experiment that he had to prevent students from "escaping" from the experimenter-constructed jail at the school.

Forget that at least one student had a psychotic break, others had medical consequences and who knows what else. Zimbardo claimed he adequately debriefed everyone at the end of the experiment and went dancing off into the sunshine of his professorship. OK, Phil, but what about the neighbors who were also involved in seeing students handcuffed at their homes and pushed into police cars or the long-term consequences of PTSD which, I'm sure, there were? How has that played out for you? Still have an absolutely guilt-free conscience about all of this? I won't go into your experiment into hypnosis which was described in a Sunday NYT magazine article years ago.

While we're at it, consider the Dr. Stanley Milgram "Obedience to Authority" experiment at Yale. He subjected naive people (call them experimental subjects) to thinking they'd killed someone with an electric shock. Women's results were tossed from the experiments because Milgram felt they provided results that weren't in line with his thinking. Oh, yes, all of this was done to see whether ordinary people could be induced to kill someone a la the Nazis during WWII. The work came directly out of that era. Milgram debriefed the subjects later and showed them they hadn't killed anyone, but what of the woman who shouted at her husband that he was no better than Eichmann? Remember Adolph Eichman who signed the travel orders to send Jews to the gas chambers?

What a wonderful legacy psychology has. I thought we'd learned but there appears to have been inadequate attention paid to psychologists' mistakes and their casual dismissal of questionable experiments. No, I didn't mention the experiment where students were actually injected with adrenaline.

I've heard of some pretty egregious behavior on the part of psychologists and psychiatrists, but the current CIA report indicates we've hit a new low with incredible rewards for the perpetrators of this tawdriness. None of the questionable work that preceded it justifies this in any way, nor am I trying to offer anything other than examples of how psychologists failed those who came to them to help in research.

I remember being in a graduate program where we were required to volunteer (not really the right word, but they used it anyway) for 10 hours of experiments in order to pass our course. There was a large board listing all of the requirements to get into each experiment and also what would disqualify you. I looked for everything that said "no paid" and allowed people wearing glasses. I did my 10 hours in boring memory experiments run by doctoral students and I know they must have wanted to pull their hair out. I was not a willing subject and they knew it.

So, how do you get honest responses from people who are being forced, coerced or tortured (as in the case of the CIA)? You don't.

Chapter 41:
Digitally Illiterate
But Able to Learn

The digital age has been around long enough for most of us to be at least minimally acquainted with the lingo, but apparently that isn't so. I had a telling illustration of this today via a chance interaction in a store. Allow me to expound on this.

While waiting for my package to be prepared, I overheard a conversation between an elderly man and the man behind the counter. The store is one of those that provide not only shipping services, but fax preparation, computers for preparing short documents and assorted tools to prepare small booklets. It's a great all-in-one spot for some people, but for others it is a place of confusion no matter the efforts to help.

I heard the discussion as the man was first directed to the correct paper weight for his intended use (he had selected a too-heavy stock for a laser printer), then a blank look came over his face and that of the guy behind the counter. What caused this absolute lack of connection?

The man had written a book some years ago, had it printed at this shop and now wanted to revise it. Simple, right? No, not simple at all. Receiving no solution for his quandary, he wheeled on his heel and began to head for the door as I stepped forward. Never having been a Girl Scout I am, nevertheless, willing to offer help when I can. I thought I might be able to help him.

I began with a simple question. "What is it that you want to do with your book?" He looked at me as thought I had just broken into his home, but stopped and briefly explained he wanted to revise his book. "They're telling me that I have to scan all the pages and then revise it, but I can't do that." My next question was pretty elementary. "What type of software are you using?"

"Software? I don't know anything about that." I explored a bit more. "What digital format is your book in and what do you want to do with it? Perhaps make it into an ebook?"

"Now you're way over my head," he explained with no hint of a smile on his face. "I don't know what scanning it is or how to scan it. I don't know what to do." I tried to offer some suggestions about how his dilemma might be resolved but he wouldn't hear any of it. His mind was made up. He lived in this world of computerized activity and he didn't even know what "digital" meant.

"I guess I'll just have to go back and retype the entire thing," he sighed. Well, yeah, I guess that's what he'll have to do and he probably won't do it with word processing software and there will be no digital footprint for his next go-round. His work will be an exercise in frustration (constantly revising entire pages on a typewriter) with a hefty dose of anger thrown in for this infernal thing called "documents" and the Internet and things digital.

I can understand how he must have felt. My suggestions were of no use to him and he left with his ream of 20 pound white paper under his arm with a bit of an angry scowl on his face. He had been undone in his literary efforts by those in charge of the world; the coders, the digital literati and a bunch of kids. It was an impossible situation for him and I can imagine the beating that typewriter was going to receive once he got back to it.

I'd been naive enough to think that everyone knew how to use a computer and was at least minimally conversant with word processing software. I didn't expect expertise in Excel, PowerPoint, Twitter, YouTube or, heaven forbid, computer coding. The light bulb went off in my head and now I understand why the local senior centers are presenting basic courses in computer use and these courses are so painfully simplistic. It was simple because they didn't know anything about computers. Digital was entirely new and unknown to them.

Some were even afraid to turn a computer on because they thought they'd break it or it would jump forward and expect them to give all sorts of elaborate commands and they were afraid of computers. Yes, afraid. They also felt inadequate and unable to learn this "stuff my gran kids know all about."

My website does have a page on Computers where I point people to some simple programs that can be helpful. One of the best places, in my estimation, is YouTube where you can learn just about anything you need to know. The problem is breaking through that fear connection.

OK, seniors, you conquered cars without heaters or oil filters, you clipped coupons to get meat during WWII, you converted from gas lights to electricity and you got a checking account. You CAN learn some basic computer operations. Sure, it's effortful and maybe it's even a bit like learning a foreign language, but just because you're over 70 or so doesn't mean your brain has been put into cold storage. You can learn and learning will really increase your sense of mastery and even self-esteem.

I guess you could say I'm asking that you show a bit of bravery in this battle of the brains, but you will be rewarded. Learning to read opened worlds of wonder for you when you first went to elementary school and the computer will do that and more. It isn't a tool for storing recipes. I remember when that was how they pitched computers to women. Recipes? The computer is a time machine with more promise and wonder than I could ever explain to anyone.

Need a GED because you never finished high school because you had to go to work to help support your family? You can do it on the Internet. Thinking of taking a vacation, but you need some ideas about where you might go, what it would cost and whether or not you'd like it? Yes, again, the Internet is there waiting like some genie in a box for your commands. And the commands are real simple, mostly "Enter" and "Copy and paste." Go for it and be amazed.

Senior citizen doesn't mean it's all over and behind you. The wonder is waiting. Take the first step.

Chapter 42: A Lesson From The Joan Rivers Playbook

Joan Rivers, the ultimate comedy performer, has left us with wonderful memories and for that and more we can all be grateful. But more than her comedy, Joan showed us that there were things we all could do in our lives. Believe it or not, she led by example.

Sure, we all know about the terrible heatbreaks she experienced and I'm not going to enumerate them here. If you know anything about Joan Rivers you've read all about them and that's sufficient. But there were things that have been revealed about her that we can all use in our daily lives to make them better in many ways. I'm not just talking about her wonderful charity and kindness to friends and strangers or her work with God's Love We Deliver (remember they've named their new Soho bakery in NYC after her) or so many other acts of kindness. She was a kind person in her life and many who never knew about it will, I'm sure, will be touched by that wonderful quality of this woman.

What I'm talking about here is her ability to see that it's not what people think of you, but what you do for you. Not in a selfish way, but in a reasonable way. She's not the first entertainer who took home a doggy bag for either herself or her dogs. One woman makes it no secret that she brings plastic containers to her meals so that she can be sure she gets all she paid for. And isn't that what we're talking about here? Getting what you paid for? Why should you send anything you can use to the scrap heap? Doesn't make sense and Joan knew that.

She also knew that a woman likes to look her best and her daughter, Melissa, knew that, too. Hair and make-up were brought into the private hospital room where she spent her final hours. Even when preparing to leave this world, Joan, like any woman, wanted to have her hair looking good. Anyone who doesn't appreciate that has to look into their hearts and find out why they would deny it to a any woman. I've only heard that remark once in my life and I hope to never hear it again. It is cruel and thoughtless. We know a woman's hair is her crowning glory, so why would you take it away in that final stage of life? It could be the final act of kindness you show and wouldn't you want that for someone you love?

Now, let's take it a step further. If hair (and perhaps make-up) are important in a woman's life, why don't hair dressers encourage women to learn how to do their own hair at home? You shouldn't have to run out to get an appointment when you need to do your hair the way your stylist does. At best, you will never match their skills, but in a pinch, you could do a pretty passable job of it.

Time to change things. Next time you go to have your hair styled or cut, why can't you have a friend stand by with a cell phone and video it so you know exactly how to comb or blow dry it? You've paying for it, aren't you? Is this a state secret you're asking them to reveal? Why don't they ever suggest making a video or is the money too much of a disincentive? I wouldn't be too keen on any stylist who refused this request. After all, they are still going to get my business, but I may need a little help myself sometime.

Same thing with make-up. Who has the time to figure out how to do your make-up and what products to use to best effect? When someone does really good make-up, why can't you video it and take a shot of all the products you'll need? This isn't Queen Victoria's time when her obstetricians were said to hide the forceps they used to deliver her children, you know. Of course, this was all because they wanted to protect the queen's privacy, you understand, not to keep all the business for themselves with their wondrous new instruments.

OK, so a lesson from The Joan Rivers' Playbook seems like a good thing. Sorry, Melissa, if you find this item a little crass, but I think your mom would have approved.

By Dr. Patricia Farrell on September 7, 2014.

Canonical link

Exported from Medium on March 17, 2025.

Chapter 43: Just a Pen, Not a Payment

Medicine is a lot of things these days. It is a science and an art at the same time, but it's also a business and an opportunity. The latter two aspects of this profession, or as one elderly physician I know says it is a "calling," provide a dilemma for some and a bit of extra cash for others.

No doubt about it, ethics plays a big role here and some of the major forces in medicine have tried to address the touchy problem of ethics. Limits have been placed on just how expensive those nifty little gifts to newly minted physicians can be and what can be accepted in good conscience. But, as in any legal document, there's wiggle room for interpretation. How do you interpret not accepting cash gifts, but allow "funds are distributed to recipients without specific attribution to sponsors." So, giving away some money but don't say who gave it? But doesn't that still mean it came from some sponsors of such programs and doesn't that have a halo effect on every sponsor participating?

In prior years, I was bemused as the young medical students who were about to graduate whooped and hollered when they saw the shiny stethoscopes, the textbooks, the pens, the tablets, even the software. It was like Christmas in late Spring for them and they delighted in it. Some, with rather grim countenances, announced that they were giving it all to the local healthcare clinic. They were in the minority of the group merriment. Others just delighted in all of it. So this was what medicine was about to give them. It was wonderful. Sure, that was years ago and, sure, things have changed.

I have worked at several hospitals and healthcare settings over the years and I've also sat in waiting rooms both as a patient and a member of a research team. The waiting room experiences are familiar to anyone who has watched the detail (aka sales persons) come and quickly be ushered into the office.

On some occasions, the person (used to be men, now it's shapely, well dressed young women) would be carrying expensive textbooks or small pieces of computer equipment. On others, the salesperson was followed by one or two men carrying large trays of steaming foods for a lunchtime presentation to the staff. Education, after all, is necessary in medicine and staff training is essential. But it's also nice to have someone pay for your lunch as you sit quietly and watch them run through their slide presentations.

Some jobs I've had allowed me to see physicians sneaking out (yes, sneaking out) of the office to give presentations of prepared slides to physicians and other healthcare workers. Last time I questioned one, he got $1,500 for each of his efforts—all while he was receiving his salary as a full-time employee at an agency. I only know because I had to help him figure out how to use a USB drive on a computer. But is he any different from the psychiatrist who held five full-time jobs (all at the same time) at various facilities? Or the other psychiatrist who signed in at one job, went to another full-time job and then, at the end of the day, went to the other to sign out? Of course, he's retired now and left instructions that he was to have no forwarding address provided to anyone.

Now a physician who has also seen the underbelly in its unattractive presentation has provided another look at medicine from his perspective. You can read it in "Doctored: The Disillusionment of an American Physician" if you wish. In it, according to reviewers, is an often unpalatable view of profiteering, cronyism, unnecessary testing and generally reprehensible behavior on the part of those who have sworn to do no harm.

Again, there's that tricky little word play. Doing "no harm" to whom or what? Do they harm the patient or society as a whole when they order unnecessary, very expensive testing that the rest of us will pay for? How about "no harm" if a patient is exposed time and time again to potentially harmful x-rays or other radiation? Well, I'll let one reviewer, from the Yale School of Medicine respond when they wrote that (the book) is "a fantastic tour through the seedy underworld of American medicine." Enough said on that account.

A physician I respect once told me that he had breakfast each morning on a regular basis with peers at a major hospital. One of the peers is an orthopedic surgeon who, when he was leaving the table, would regularly joke, "Well, got to be off to do another unnecessary surgery." He was joking, surely. What's the standing joke in medicine about surgeons? Go to a surgeon and you get surgery. Do they imply that you get it whether you need it or not? Oh, no, can't be true.

What's the remedy for all of this? Tighter control by someone or some agency? Doesn't always work because of the lobbying that's involved and we consumer have no lobbyists to speak of. Hospitals should ride rough shod on fast-and-loose physicians? Not when they're the ones who bring in all the money and funds all those extensive building projects. Will the new trend of hiring physicians away from private practice and making them hospital employees help? Do you think so?

All it comes down to is caveat emptor as it does when you buy anything. You're buying or paying for a service and you have a right to negotiate, get a second opinion or begin a grassroots movement against anything you see needs fixing. Yes, it's left on your already-burdened shoulders.

Chapter 44: Brain Cleaning? Is That Something We Should Be Doing?

We clean our clothes, we clean our homes, and we clean out our file cabinets, but do we ever think about cleaning out our brains?

Researchers are very concerned about neurodegenerative diseases due to their devastation. The research has been ongoing for many decades. While some advances have been made in the discovery of certain substances that may lead to negative brain changes, we are still searching for that elusive answer.

One of the main questions being asked is what causes the brain to be unable to clear itself of metabolic byproducts from brain activity. In other words, it's like, what do you do with the "garbage" that is left over, and if you do nothing, is that what is causing the problem?

This direction appears to be the most promising track being pursued by research in understanding how the brain naturally attempts to clean itself and what might be inhibiting this process—one of the factors may be aging. However, what actions can we take to facilitate this clearing process, given that aging is a natural part of life? Can we facilitate this clearing process in some way, despite a person's natural aging?

The cleaning process is essential if your brain continues to function optimally. Alzheimer's disease, one of the disorders associated with decreased brain function and cleaning, is one of our most feared diseases.

Some of the most significant signs of Alzheimer's disease are widespread amyloid plaques and neurofibrillary tangles. Neurons, white matter, and synapses — those tiny areas where all intercellular action takes place — often accompany these abnormal changes. It's still not clear what causes these neuropathological changes, but it's likely that both genetic and environmental factors play a role. But that does not diminish our having hope that certain activities now or in the future will be effective in protecting our brains.

As we age, our brains have a harder time removing cellular waste that accumulates and damages brain cells. The glymphatic system and the meningeal lymphatic system are two systems that work together to remove waste. The brain uses the glymphatic system, which doesn't have any blood vessels, to get rid of cellular waste products and soluble waste proteins. As time passes, this system becomes increasingly vulnerable.

Findings that show less glymphatic clearance in aging brains indicate that both the rate of cerebrospinal fluid formation (we constantly produce cerebrospinal fluid, which must be used and then eliminated) and the rate of change slow down as people age.

Major health problems happen in the brain when this system stops working properly. This slowing down of waste removal allows amyloid-beta and tau proteins to build up, which causes neuroinflammation and neurotoxicity. Neuroinflammation, in fact, is not only implicated in Alzheimer's disease but most probably involved in numerous mental disorders.

After all is said and done, we are making headway, but there are no hacks, no magic formulas, no secrets - simply basic things we can do every day to help ourselves and keep our brains healthy. You might already be practicing You might already be practicing these habits, but you may not have recognized the true benefits of activities like exercising once a day or even three times a week.

A small experimental sample has discovered that there may be an opportunity for medical devices on the skin's surface to remove some waste. The technique is called massaging, but it is too early to know if this will be a radical breakthrough that can be utilized by many of us. Currently, researchers are only exploring it with animal models.

Let's outline some of the things that researchers are recommending you consider in your plan to clean your brain and reward yourself with renewed cognition and life.

According to research on brain waste clearance, the following ways have been shown to *improve the glymphatic system's function* in humans:

A National Institute of Health study reveals that the glymphatic system functions optimally during sleep, when the brain eliminates waste proteins. This means that the *length and quality of deep sleep should be a top priority*. Surprisingly, during sleep, the brain undergoes changes that act like a "washing machine" for waste to be efficiently removed, making sleep a vital component of this entire process.

1. **Sleep**: To achieve quality sleep, people should aim to get between 7 and 9 hours of sleep every night. Professional institutes suggest that sleeping on your side is the best position

for improved glymphatic clearance, as it may help your body eliminate waste more efficiently.

2. **Lifestyle Choices**: Engaging in physical activity helps to alter glymphatic clearance and support vascular health in the brain, which is beneficial for the brain's waste removal system.

3. Changes to the **Diet**: Omega-3 fatty acids are beneficial for the brain because they impact glymphatic clearance, aiding in the brain's waste removal. Studies have shown that partial fasting enables the body to eliminate waste more effectively.

4. Limiting **Alcohol**: Drinking too much alcohol impairs the glymphatic clearing process.

5. Reduce **Stress**: Long-term stress hinders the brain's ability to eliminate waste.

6. Monitor Your **Blood Pressure**: For the glymphatic system to function properly, blood pressure must be under control, and arterial health must be optimal.

Now that we understand the importance of cleaning our minds and how we can support this natural process, we have the tools needed to help ourselves. As always, each of us must decide what, when, and how much we do.

You don't need to hire a cleaning service because everything is at your disposal and within your discretion.

Chapter 45: Simple Isometric Exercises to Build Strength and Mental Wellness for All Ages

Each day, while engaging in your usual activities, you can incorporate exercise into your routine, which will provide many benefits to you.

Isometric exercises are ideal for incorporating into your routines, as they involve engaging muscles without moving the joints. These exercises can be easily incorporated into day-to-day activities and offer benefits to individuals of all ages, improving both their physical and mental health.

In fact, isometric workouts are an excellent starting point for a healthier lifestyle because they require minimal resistance and can be performed at a lower intensity. As you become more self-assured, comfortable, and stronger, you can integrate more isotonic motions and weighted exercises, both of which are great ways to build strength and confidence. What are some ways isometrics can improve your body and mind?

1. Helps to preserve the strength of joints

Isometric exercises are more effective than traditional strength training in strengthening joints. Additionally, they can accomplish this without experiencing the discomfort commonly associated with other movements.

2. Causes a decrease in high blood pressure

An investigation conducted in 2023 showed that isometric workouts, particularly the wall squat, have the potential to be an efficient method for lowering blood pressure. By holding a squat position while leaning your back and shoulders on a wall behind you, you can do an isometric leg workout known as a wall squat (also known as a wall sit). The mechanism by which this workout affects blood pressure is not fully understood by researchers; however, they believe it may be related to the blood flow into and out of muscles when they contract and release.

In a study published in October 2023 in the British Journal of Sports Medicine, researchers combined the results of 270 clinical trials involving over 15,000 participants. The effects of exercise on blood pressure were documented in each of the experiments, which lasted for a minimum of two weeks.

Exercising in various ways helped lower blood pressure, as expected. Isometric exercise training has been proven to be the most effective form of exercise, particularly for individuals with high blood pressure.

The pain associated with osteoarthritis can be excruciating, particularly when the joint is being moved through its full range of motion or when the patient is exercising. Individuals with osteoarthritis may benefit from engaging in isometric exercises to activate their muscles and maintain strength before adding additional resistance. This method is effective in reducing discomfort, increasing the range of motion, and enhancing function, according to research. How long should these muscles be held for the best results?

Beginners should hold for 3-10 seconds; experienced individuals, 30+ seconds. Cleveland Clinic Health Essentials suggests a gradual increase in exercise hold time, based on your body's feedback and increasing strength.

Here are some isometric exercises. Remember to discuss this with your healthcare provider before any exercise and begin slowly — do not attempt to proceed faster than your body can handle the exercise. Everyone will progress at their own pace.

1. **Phone calls and push-ups.**

You should position yourself so that you are an arm's length away from a wall and rest your palms flat against it at shoulder height. This should be done when you are standing and talking on the phone or waiting in line. Maintain this position while leaning forward slightly and engaging the muscles in your chest, shoulders, and core. This exercise helps ease stress and anxiety while also strengthening the upper body and improving posture.

2. **Planks at the desk**

By placing your hands on the edge of your desk and walking your feet back until your body forms a straight line, you may turn your desk into a useful tool for increasing your fitness level. This modified plank position should be held for thirty to sixty seconds.

In addition to preventing the detrimental consequences of sitting for extended periods, this workout targets the entire core, as well as the shoulders and arms. Besides removing mental fog and boosting attention throughout the workday, the concentration required to maintain good form serves as a form of mindfulness.

3. Commute glute squeezes

In any situation, whether you are sitting at your desk, in a car, or on public transportation, you can subtly clench your glute muscles and hold the contraction for ten to fifteen seconds before releasing it. As you perform this exercise, you will strengthen the largest muscle group in your body while also preventing the muscle weakness that can result from prolonged sitting. A meditative pattern can be created through the repetitive nature of squeeze-and-release, which helps reduce stress caused by commuting and promotes mental peace.

4. Calf Raises While Carrying Out Daily Tasks

Raise yourself up onto your toes and maintain the position for a few seconds before gradually lowering yourself back down when doing tasks like brushing your teeth, cooking, or doing the dishes. By strengthening the calves and improving circulation in the lower legs, this exercise is particularly beneficial for individuals who spend a significant amount of time sitting or standing for extended periods.

5. Abdominal Support During the Day

This invisible exercise involves gently drawing your navel toward your spine and maintaining that contraction while breathing normally throughout any activity you engage in. This is something you should practice while walking, sitting in meetings, or performing household or work duties.

A consistent abdominal bracing routine helps develop the deep core muscles, which improve posture and support spinal health. In addition to enhancing bodily awareness, the conscious link between the mind and core muscles can also serve as a point of anchoring for maintaining presence and reducing stress throughout the day.

Isometrics are a wonderful way to incorporate simple exercises into your daily routine, eliminating the need to go to the gym, use equipment, or take time out of your day. Each day includes exercise, allowing you to reap the benefits while going about your normal activities.

Chapter 46: Why Scientists Want You to Use Your Other Hand

Hand dominance may provide brain resources that you were previously unaware of or enhance the ones you already possess.

When my mother entered elementary school, she was left-handed, but the school viewed that as a deficit. What do you suppose they did? Yes, she told me they tied her left hand behind her back so that she was forced to use her right hand.

Left-handedness has long posed a challenge in many cultures, as nearly everything has been designed for right-handed individuals. I also have a relative who is left-handed, and the school saw no issues in that regard. He was an excellent student, graduated with top grades, and went on to a professional school where he had to use specialized instruments. The issue? Most of the instruments were, once again, designed for right-handed users.

He struggled significantly to find left-handed instruments, and he wasn't alone. I also had a friend who was left-handed and enjoyed playing golf. Most golf equipment is similarly designed for right-handed players. Again, he faced difficulty finding left-handed golf clubs. But one time, he had a great chuckle when someone stole his golf clubs from the trunk of his car. "I wonder how surprised they're going to be when they find out they can't use those clubs because they're made for a left-handed golfer," He said with a glorious smile on his face.

Have you ever tried using your opposite hand to perform your daily activities? Do you believe that training your non-dominant hand can open up new creative channels or stimulate old, dormant brain regions? Recent studies indicate that the benefits of non-dominant hand training might be more useful than previously thought, yet more complex.

Have you ever thought about what would happen if you started using your "other" hand for everyday activities? Perhaps you have heard claims that training your non-dominant hand can unlock hidden creativity or tap into unused parts of your brain. The reality is more complex than these claims, but recent research has provided some intriguing insights into what happens when we try to use our non-dominant hand.

What the Science Shows

The idea that using your non-dominant hand will suddenly make you more creative is largely a myth. As researchers have found, while blogs and self-help articles often promise dramatic cognitive boosts, the scientific evidence tells a different story. Any improvements you gain will likely be specific to the skills you practice, rather than providing a general creativity enhancement.

Actual Changes in Your Brain

When you persistently train your non-dominant hand, measurable changes occur in your brain. Studies using advanced brain imaging have shown that sustained practice with your non-dominant hand creates new neural pathways and strengthens existing ones. This process, called neuroplasticity, demonstrates your brain's remarkable ability to adapt and reorganize itself.

For example, research on precision drawing with the non-dominant hand revealed increased functional connectivity among various brain regions involved in hand control and movement planning. Similarly, studies on learning to use chopsticks (granted, most of us rarely use chopsticks) with the non-dominant hand showed significant changes in brain activity patterns after just a few weeks of practice.

A Possible Schedule to Use

The following is based on research in this area, but it serves as a simple and potential guide for anyone who wants to test some of the research theories. This is not a specific training program for anyone but a more recreational activity. Remember that research always has imperfections, and some of these results are due to the samples used, the areas where it was conducted, and the researcher's own biases.

Training your non-dominant hand requires a structured approach, which begins with fundamental skills before advancing. If you think you will be turned into a Picasso or a best-selling author because of these exercises, you may be disappointed. There was only one Picasso, but you can possibly improve some things for yourself. Exactly what they will be is undefined and unknown. *Daily practice of 15–20 minutes may lead to enhanced abilities.*

Start with the basics (Weeks 1–2)

Write your name slowly with your non-dominant hand, followed by practicing the alphabet and basic words. The initial appearance of your writing does not need to be perfect. Back to that time in elementary school when you were first learning your alphabet and how your handwriting had to be improved by repeatedly drawing circles and then letters. Using the non-dominant hand will be very much like the initial learning. This is the handwriting part of your exercise.

Now, draw basic shapes, including circles and lines, while concentrating on maintaining control rather than achieving perfection. The initial exercises help your brain learn fundamental motor patterns, which serve as a foundation.

Move into daily life (Weeks 3–4)

After gaining control of your writing movements, begin using your non-dominant hand for basic everyday activities. Begin by using your non-dominant hand to hold your coffee cup and use a spoon to eat during meals, starting with basic foods.

Do not attempt these tasks while using hot liquids or foods in your non-dominant hand. We don't want anyone to have an unpleasant experience. So, care is the watchword here. Spend daily intervals with your computer mouse positioned on the opposite side of your normal use. This technique helps you connect your practice sessions to actual, real-world applications.

Refine your skills (Weeks 5–8)

Progress to performing more accurate tasks with your non-dominant hand. The activities you should attempt next include threading needles, using scissors for basic cuts, and brushing your teeth. Add creative elements too—drawing, painting, or playing instruments if you have them.

Master advanced coordination (Week 9+)

The last step involves performing complex tasks that will push your abilities to their limits. The brain development process benefits significantly from learning to use chopsticks, while activities like playing catch and writing whole paragraphs integrate all your learned skills.

Progressively incorporate your non-dominant hand into your hobbies, cooking activities, and problem-solving tasks. But always proceed cautiously with every activity in which you will engage.

Will this program work for you? Only you can make that determination, and you are also the one who will decide whether you want to engage in this activity. It might be interesting, it might be useful, or it might be something you decide to toss aside. No harm.

Chapter 47: A Simple Touch Technique That's Backed by Multiple Studies

We know that touch is effective in some forms of therapy, and now we're examining another form that may be even more potent than we previously thought.

I've seen people, deep in thought, tapping their front teeth lightly with their fingertips, and I never gave it much thought. I also once had a doctoral student working on a dissertation about a type of therapy that involved tapping, and I always wondered how strong the research evidence was for it.

Could a few gentle taps here and there help ease tension, aches, and pains? The science underlying Emotional Freedom Technique

(EFT) tapping is robust, despite its unconventional nature. Evidence suggests that EFT tapping can be effective in addressing several issues. What are they? They range from anxiety and phobias to depression and post-traumatic stress disorder (PTSD), insomnia, pain, and even athletic performance, according to a meta-analysis of 50 studies published in 2022.

The emergence of this new type of therapy aligns with other therapeutic approaches. We have seen that it depends on some form of physical change. For example, EMDR relies on changing the direction of our eyes. We have to wonder what connection is made between the eyes and the mind, and that hugely complex conglomeration of cells in our brains. To us, it seems so simple, and yet it is too complex for us to even attempt to explain. What does the theory indicate happens, and what are the concerns about this specific therapy?

EMDR (Eye Movement Desensitization and Reprocessing) represents a structured therapy that assists people in recovering from traumatic experiences and disturbing life events. The person recalls distressing memories during EMDR sessions through brief recollections while following the therapist's hand movements, sounds, or taps that move from left to right. The bilateral stimulation process in EMDR therapy theoretically helps the brain transform traumatic memories into less intense emotional experiences that become easier to handle.

The brain mechanisms involved in EMDR therapy operate similarly to those that occur during REM sleep, when the brain naturally processes emotional memories. The therapeutic environment enables the brain to reorganize its memory storage and response mechanisms for painful experiences, thereby facilitating healing. However, while this is an assumption, we have no evidence that the brain actively reorganizes thoughts. Are we exploring the body mechanisms that may be activated during acupuncture therapy, but differently?

EFT and Where to Tap

Emotional Freedom Technique is based on the seemingly absurd premise that tapping on specific points on the body (such as the collarbone or eyebrow) will alleviate tension and pain. This comprehensive method requires no specialized equipment and can be performed independently at any time and from any location.

In this technique, you concentrate on a single thought or feeling by tapping on certain areas of your body (mostly your head and face). Think of it as a combination of current psychology with acupressure sites to alleviate stress and improve mood, anxiety, and discomfort.

Using acupoints as a starting point, EFT tapping emerged in the 1970s and 1980s. The twelve main meridians (channels) that distribute energy throughout the body are outlined in TCM. Along these meridians, acupoints are located, and they can be activated through acupressure or acupuncture.

Over 100 peer-reviewed studies, meta-analyses, and outcome reviews demonstrate the effectiveness of EFT for psychological and physiological indications. EFT provides a simple learning process for application while being non-pharmacological, cost-free, and purportedly safe for stress and anxiety reduction and burnout symptom management.

What Is the Procedure?

Step one involves tapping on certain areas of the body while reciting a selected phrase. A practitioner will tap patients when administering the treatment.

EFT Tapping Points (in order):

□•□Karate Chop Point (Side of Hand)

□Location: Outer edge of the hand, below the pinky finger.

□What's Done: Tapped with fingertips of the opposite hand while stating a setup phrase (e.g., "Even though I feel anxious, I deeply and completely accept myself.")

□•□Eyebrow Point (EB)

□Location: Where the eyebrow begins, nearest to the bridge of the nose.

□What's Done: Gently tap with two fingers; often the first point after the setup. Focus on the emotional intensity.

□•□Side of Eye (SE)

□Location: On the bone beside the outer corner of the eye.

□What's Done: Tap lightly with two fingers; helps reduce stress and anxiety.

□•□Under Eye (UE)

□Location: On the bone directly under the eye.

□What's Done: Tapped to help release fear and physical tension.

□•□Under Nose (UN)

□Location: Between the nose and the upper lip.

□What's Done: Tapped to address shame, guilt, and powerlessness.

□•□Chin Point (CP)

□Location: Midway between the bottom lip and the chin, in the indentation.

□What's Done: Tap to reduce embarrassment and indecision.

□•□Collarbone Point (CB)

□Location: Just below the collarbone, slightly toward the center of the chest.

□What's Done: Tapped to balance the body and release generalized anxiety.

□•□Under Arm (UA)

□Location: About 4 inches below the armpit, in line with the nipple.

□What's Done: Tap to help release emotional baggage and promote calm.

□•□Top of Head (TH)

□Location: Crown of the head, center point.

□What's Done: Tapped to reinforce emotional release and integrate the calming effects.

Each point is tapped 5–7 times, usually while repeating a reminder phrase linked to the emotion or problem being addressed (e.g., "this fear," "this tightness in my chest"). The complete sequence is executed multiple times until a change in emotional or physical distress becomes noticeable.

Research about EFT benefits for stress management, anxiety relief, and burnout reduction continues to grow through documented studies. The available research shows EFT functions as an effective self-help method, and healthcare professionals and students can use it in their practice.

The American Psychological Association's Division 12 Task Force on Empirically Validated Treatments evaluated these studies. Numerous investigations have studied the psychological impacts of EFT. But existing research lacks sufficient studies about the physical effects of EFT on the body. What does it do and how does it work? That part is still to be answered.

Is this therapy as powerful and valuable as it is being presented? It may help individuals with specific issues, but the jury is still out on how it works. Additionally, there have been complaints from some patients that it made their symptoms worse, others who state it didn't help at all, and still others who found it helpful.

But haven't we heard that about many therapies from patients? It may have more to do with patient expectations, beliefs in more traditional methods, and the individual involved with the patients (if not a self-help form of EFT). As always, caveat emptor.

Chapter 48: The Productive and Powerful "Crumb Method" of Writing Creatively and Smart

Story ideas are all around — start using the methods of famous writers.

Writing is an exploration. You start from nothing and learn as you go. — E. L. Doctorow

Writing is what you want to do and what you enjoy doing for the most part. But there are too many instances when a writer faces a void in their production, and that's where my theory of the "Crumb Method" comes in. Where did it come from?

Conferences, whether on writing or anything else, can be so boring and disappointing that you wonder why you attended. You had hoped that some spark of insight, a fresh approach, something—anything—would be offered to fire up your writing imagination and engine. You were wrong. At least, that's the way you felt when you left.

My friend, that's where you missed those valuable parts hidden—the ones you overlooked because of boredom. It happens to everyone.

I recall one famous writer, Isaac Asimov, and another whose name I can't remember giving me writing advice. Asimov said, to paraphrase, "I can't write about something that someone else hasn't written on before me." He admitted he needed other writers' creativity to fire up his own and to set him on a path.

The other writer admitted he "stole" everything he could from other writers. Of course, he didn't plagiarize, but he got his ideas and maybe his style or his genre from other writers; I'll never know. Remember, you don't have to keep reinventing the wheel.

You can aim to write "It was the best of times, it was the worst of times…" in terms of today's world, and you don't have to be Charles Dickens to do so. Do we live in two different times now? Read the newspapers, and there are the ideas you are seeking, just as Dickens probably did.

Where are the creative crumbs?

Since I originally wrote this article, I have had over 40 flash fiction stories accepted for publication. All of them were inspired by places I've been, people to whom I've spoken, or things I have observed.

Everything was turned into complete stories that rang true for editors at publications.

Once again, I have had an epiphany regarding a flash fiction story that I have written. While watching a recent film, one scene depicted a machine cleaning a star on the Hollywood Walk of Fame.

It opened my eyes to a new beginning to the story that I am writing. So, I will now come out of my comfort zone and begin writing in a voice I rarely use, and I think it will improve the story and strengthen its appeal.

Even when I've had a rejection, there have been encouraging comments. One editor thought the story should be turned into a novel. Of course, I feel my genre is in flash fiction and short stories—novels are not for me. I may occasionally enjoy reading one, but the form isn't a comfortable one for me. This coming May (2023), I will have another flash story (Courtesy Never Dies) in a university publication (Woodcrest Magazine).

Yes, I have others (about 10 of them) in various stages of being written. In that, I follow Isaac Asimov's example of always having something of interest about which to write. They are all waiting for me. All of the stories I wrote in my flash fiction book, Unexpected Short Tales of Surprise, were sparked by things I saw, things I had been told or ideas that came from watching someone. The book is now featured on Apple Books and Kobo.

How did I come across what I saw as a mind-opening experience? I had to attend a seminar that was required to maintain my license. I didn't want to go, but I had no choice.

The presenters began with the usual PowerPoint slides and droned on. But as I listened, I heard a word that was unusual to me. I wrote it down in my small notebook and decided it had a grain, or a crumb, that would spark an idea for an article.

Once I returned home, I began researching the term and decided I could write an article on it. I sent it to a professional journal only to be told they wanted to publish it, but I had to have an MD co-author.

I contacted a friend who gave me the name and number of an MD in the area, and I told her all she had to do was read it and agree to be co-author; no writing was required. If you know anything about medicine, publishing is king, and getting an article in a major journal is a great accomplishment. And when you don't even have to write anything, how could it get any better?

The Crumb Method was born at that seminar, and I've used it ever since. Oh, BTW, they published the article, and I began to receive offers to appear on TV shows. It opened up a whole new area for me. I was also invited to join a professional entertainment union, which meant I got paid for my appearances. And it all started at a seminar I didn't want to attend.

Listening with the "third ear"

Psychologists—I'm one—are taught to use their third ear in therapy sessions. Simply put, it means you listen for what isn't being said; it provides information to explore further.

Anyone can train themselves to use this technique and apply it to the Crumb Method for writing purposes. Any conversation, a situation on the street, TV show, a news broadcast, or anything that you hear or read can contain that crumb you're seeking. Perhaps eavesdropping isn't polite, but you have to use all the tools at your disposal, and this is one of them.

Begin your training right now. See if you can find one word or phrase that holds the key to something you'll write. It's there. Write it down and start thinking about how you will utilize it.

Chapter 49: For I Was Hungry, and You Gave Me Food: Food insecurity and AI's hope for the future

Food insecurity is not something with which I am only intellectually familiar. I knew it in my early childhood when we lived in a cold-water flat owned by the local slumlord. My mom tried valiantly to feed us and went for cooking classes at the local social services office.

Food selection was a major topic in the classes, as was how to handle little in the way of money.

My mother, like so many others in our neighborhood, went without food in order to feed us. The woman downstairs tried to subsist on adulterated black coffee and cigarettes; the milk was for her five children.

When news of "cheap meat" hit the local gossip mill, it ran through the neighborhood like a virus, and the mothers were quick to act. I remember rushing with my mother (I was about five at the time) to the local subway. The train took us to a smelly meat wholesale market on the Lower West Side of Manhattan. Women stood in a long queue and waited patiently in the heat as the meat was brought out. It was never the bargain they had been led to believe.

Then the area was known as the Meatpacking District. Slaughterhouses lined the rail line that brought in the animals. The railheads have been replaced by flowering plants, exotic sculptures and tourists with expensive cameras and it's known as the High Line Park. Few of the market's vestiges remain on the street below. Sunbathers loll away the afternoon where animals once raised their frantic voices.

The developers had come in to scoop up the coveted Hudson River views as the wholesalers left, and the abattoir was transformed into a playground for the wealthy. Markets with their blood-drenched cobblestone streets, sides of beef on hooks, and men in stained, bloody aprons are gone.

Trendy clubs and expensive hi-rise condos have replaced the once-familiar. But my vivid memory hangs on like those sides of beef and the flies that swarmed the crowds of poor women clutching small children.

They should put up a sign like the one on NYU's building for the Triangle Shirtwaist Factory fire. This new sign should stand as a testament to the poor women who ran there for meat they could barely afford for their hungry families.

Food insecurity in a country of plenty

The term is used increasingly in the media, but what does it mean? "Food insecurity, which the US Department of Agriculture (USDA) defines as 'a household-level economic and social condition of limited or uncertain access to adequate food,' is an important national health problem and an underrecognized social determinant of health. It places a substantial burden on our society through health care and social costs. People experiencing food insecurity often consume a nutrient-poor diet, which may contribute to the development of obesity, heart disease, hypertension, diabetes, and other chronic diseases. People who live in food-insecure households also have difficulties in managing diet-related chronic conditions."

In 2018, the United States Department of Agriculture noted that the highest food insecurity rates were for single-mother households and households with incomes below the poverty line.

One in seven households with children were affected by food insecurity in 2018. The USDA also stated, "Parents often shield children from experiencing food insecurity, particularly very low food security, even when the parents themselves are food insecure... In about half of those food-insecure households with children, only the adults experienced food insecurity." The intention was, as it had been in my neighborhood, for the parents to provide food for the children at risk. Parents were willing to endure food insecurity.

Nutrition experts tell parents to provide healthy meals and snacks, fresh fruits, and vegetables for their children. How does anyone provide "healthy meals and snacks" for their children when they don't have the money to buy them?

How does anyone keep fresh fruit and vegetables in the home when there are no food markets in the area? How does any parent who cannot provide for their children feel when they are told they must?

How does anyone get a job to buy these staples when towns ensure no bus transportation for those seeking jobs? Why are sidewalks not placed along roadways for those who must walk?

All of these questions are ones to be debated at length before anyone can dare to cast aspersions at the impoverished and their children. All of the issues relate to food insecurity and a system that grinds down the underprivileged.

Where is food insecurity most acute in the US?

The USDA has supplied graphics depicting the states with regard to their food insecurity averages. Statistics provide an eye-opening picture of where food insecurity is greatest. Nothing but the graphic is needed.

The price paid for lack of nutrition

"Food insecurity and insufficiency are associated with adverse health and developmental outcomes in U.S. children. Among 6- to 12-y-old children, food insufficiency was associated with poorer mathematics scores, grade repetition, absenteeism, tardiness, visits to a psychologist, anxiety, aggression, psychosocial dysfunction, and difficulty getting along with other children. Among 15- to 16-y-old adolescents, food insufficiency was associated with depressive disorders and suicide symptoms after controlling for income and other factors."

How does the availability of popular foods in schools hinder children's ability to learn? As noted in one article, these food plans are "loaded with sugars, caffeine, chemicals, and sodium; many popular menu items are leaving kids tired, unfocused, jittery and sick," which not only impacts children's grades and performance but also influences their behavior and moods.

"... recent studies reveal that diets with high levels of saturated fats actually impair learning and memory. Unfortunately, foods with saturated fats are often the most affordable and widely available in schools. French fries, sugary desserts, cheeseburgers, chicken nuggets, and other cafeteria staples are filling kids with food that actually lowers their brainpower before sending them back to class."

School lunches, especially poorly planned and funded ones, therefore, undercut a child's ability to do well in school and in life after graduation. The lunch programs are not a reflection of what nutritionists are suggesting is required for healthy child development. Why not?

Kids never see what is happening to them and have no voice in how they are fed. Their brains will suffer the consequences of ignorance on the part of those who determine the food served and its nutritional value.

The myth that denies the hungry

One prominent myth that is mouthed too often is that of "the welfare queen," a woman on welfare who scammed the system. Her machinations were puffed up to support cutting back on programs for feeding the poor, the elderly, social services, and even children. How did it all happen?

Ronald Reagan wasn't above twisting the truth and fashioning a message that would appeal to those who supported him.

"...Reagan's soliloquies on welfare fraud are often remembered as shameless demagoguery. Many accounts report that Reagan coined the term "welfare queen" and that this woman in Chicago **was a fictional character**. In 2007, the New York Times' Paul Krugman wrote that "*the bogus story of the Cadillac-driving welfare queen [was] a gross exaggeration of a minor case of welfare fraud.*" MSNBC's Chris Matthews says the whole thing is racist malarkey—a coded reference to Black indolence and criminality designed to appeal to working-class whites."

The myth was created, and people believed it. Today, the urban myth continues as the raison d'être for denying the poor and under-privileged in our society. Shameful and false as it has been proven, it continues to infest minds.

AI and food production

Food production can have a significant impact on food insecurity in all parts of the world, and AI is bringing a new day to farming methods. A multiplicity of organizations are making worldwide attempts to address the food production of organizations and corporations. The technology is as close as a cell phone.

A new generation of apps, including Farmwave, PlantVillage, and Plantix, are using learning algorithms in a variety of ways. They diagnose plant diseases and pests in seconds rather than days or weeks and aid in food distribution and the elimination of spoilage.

The crucial shortcuts in time are estimated to increase global food production by 25–70% in 2050, and it is predicted that it will reach the ability to nourish 9–10 billion people in the next 30 years.

Machine learning tools are also being used to create what is known as "predictive ordering" (Shelf Engine), Calorie Mama, a visual food journal, and other emerging technologies to create more equitable food systems. If a nutritionist isn't available, an app is right there.

Wholesome Wave has a card-based payment platform that supports an initiative called Wholesome RX, which uses data from supermarket loyalty cards to generate coupons for nutritious foods and personalized diet recommendations. The food and vegetable prescription program is administered at participating health clinics and is used by Medicaid patients who want to eat more fresh produce.

AI is also being used in food banks around the world as well as in creating meal kits to develop and deliver nutritious meals to food-insecure families. Feeding Children Everywhere provides families in the program with 40 prepackaged, dehydrated red lentil jambalayas and apple pie oats. Primarily, this program is for working families that may not be able to go to a food bank because of work requirements.

"Emerging technologies are transforming how we produce, distribute, and consume what we eat by bringing food to people instead of bringing people to food. A new report by the Refresh Working Group featuring Food Tank, Google, the US Chamber of Commerce, and more than twenty other partners, called Refresh: Food and Tech, from Soil to Supper, highlights more than 20 digital platforms and artificial intelligence algorithms being adopted across the U.S. food supply chain by farmers, distributors, grocers, retailers, and consumers."

The world of food and food production has undergone innovation, thanks to AI, and countless individuals and families will benefit. A brighter future awaits us as more creativity is brought to bear on the AI currently in place.

But there are two stumbling blocks to this vision of a better world: politicians and the myth of the welfare queen. Can we solve both for the sake of our kids and our people, please?

Chapter 50: Monday, Monday, Anxiety Strikes and Sticks for a Lifetime

You know that sinking feeling when Sunday evening rolls around and you think about the week ahead? Or that heavy dread that settles in your chest on Monday morning before you even check your emails? You're not imagining it, and you're definitely not alone.

New scientific research reveals that Monday anxiety isn't just a cultural meme—it's a real biological phenomenon that affects millions of people worldwide. Even more fascinating? The effects of Monday stress show up in our bodies weeks after we experience it.

The Science Behind Your Monday Dread

Researchers at the University of Hong Kong studied over 3,500 adults in England 50 or older. It made a startling discovery: people who felt anxious on Mondays had 23% higher levels of the stress hormone cortisol in their hair samples collected up to two months later. There was a distinctive difference between those who had Monday anxiety and those who felt anxious on other days of the week. Reading the hair samples was all that the investigators had to do to come up with their answer.

Consider that for a moment. Your Monday anxiety doesn't just ruin your Monday—it literally changes your body's stress response for weeks afterward. What other day of the week does that to you? The answer is simple, and it isn't any other day of the week except Monday. For that reason, we need to take exceptional care of ourselves regarding how we start off the week.

The researchers used hair samples because, unlike blood or saliva tests that capture stress levels at a single moment, hair acts like a biological diary, recording hormone levels over months. What they found was clear evidence that Monday anxiety triggers something in your body's stress system that causes it to go haywire.

The researcher who led the study, Dr. Tarani Chandola, explains that this "Monday effect" was present whether people were working or retired. This would suggest that our culture's collective dread of Mondays runs so deep that even people not bound by traditional work schedules still feel it. Retiring isn't the answer, therefore, and we need to look at other things that can be helpful in responding to this cultural difficulty.

Why Mondays Hit Different

What makes Mondays uniquely awful is that it turns out there are several factors working against us:

Your Internal Clock is Confused

Most of us follow dramatically different sleep schedules on weekends. We sleep in late Saturday and Sunday, then suddenly have to wake up early Monday morning. This creates what scientists call "social jet "lag"—similar to traveling across time zones, but happening every single week. Your cortisol levels (the stress hormone, as you know) should peak before you wake up to give you energy. But as we now know, instead of that normal spike, you are getting a stress spike during your commute and throughout Monday morning, leaving you feeling off-kilter.

The Transition Shock

Your brain craves predictability and routine. While weekends offer freedom and relaxation, they also represent a complete disruption to your weekday patterns. Monday forces an abrupt shift back to structure, deadlines, and responsibilities. This transition shock activates your body's stress response, flooding your system with cortisol and adrenaline.

Anticipatory Anxiety

Often, the dread builds Sunday evening—what many call the "Sunday scaries." I'm sure you are aware of this, but you thought nobody was researching it.

What you're doing is you begin mentally reviewing your upcoming week, imagining worst-case scenarios, and feeling overwhelmed before Monday even arrives. Psychologists referred to this as "catastrophizing." This anticipatory anxiety can actually be worse than the reality of Monday itself.

Social and Work Pressures

Monday is statistically the day when we face the highest workloads, most stressful meetings, and greatest social pressures. If you're already dealing with job dissatisfaction, difficult colleagues, or feeling unfulfilled in your career, Monday becomes a weekly reminder of these larger issues.

The Real-World Impact

Monday anxiety isn't just about feeling grumpy. Research shows that Mondays are associated with:

- Higher rates of heart attacks and strokes
- Increased suicide rates, particularly among young adults
- Lower work productivity
- More sick days taken
- Higher levels of emotional stress across all age groups

The biological stress response triggered by Monday anxiety affects your immune system, blood pressure, blood sugar control, and even your heart's ability to respond to stress. It's not overly dramatic to say that chronic Monday anxiety can affect your long-term health.

We are aware of the current published research that points to Mondays being especially challenging for everyone. What can you do? One effective strategy is to prepare for Mondays in advance. Don't wait until the last minute because you know it will not work. You need to sit down calmly and think through the week ahead so that you can be prepared in advance. No one needs to have been a member of any Scouts' programs to know that preparation is everything.

Why not consider this list that may be helpful and that you can adjust however you need, because not everybody's schedule is the same? Each step needs to be tailored to your individual needs. You're in charge, as I always say, and I encourage people to think that way.

The good news? You can retrain your brain and body to respond differently to Mondays. Here are five evidence-based strategies that actually work:

1. Master Your Sleep Schedule

This is the most important change you can make. Try to keep your bedtime and wake-up time within one to two hours of your weekday schedule, even on weekends. Yes, this means less sleeping in, but it prevents the social jet lag that makes Monday mornings so brutal.

Start immediately: Set a consistent bedtime routine. Turn off devices 30 minutes before bedtime, and avoid large meals and alcohol close to sleep. If you must sleep in on weekends, limit it to one extra hour maximum. Sleep is such an important part of our life, and we now know how it can affect every aspect of our lives. We aren't just sleepy. If we don't get enough sleep, we are less motivated, less creative, and less well. It has a great effect on our immune system's efficiency.

2. Create Monday Morning Rituals You Actually Enjoy

Instead of making Monday morning about rushing to check emails and diving into stress, design a routine that gives you something to look forward to. This could be a special breakfast, your favorite podcast, a short walk outside, or even just 10 minutes of stretching.

Start this week by picking one small pleasure and commit to it every Monday morning for the next month. Maybe it is your special-occasion coffee or enjoying your favorite playlist as you get ready. It doesn't have to be a major thing in your life, just something small that will add a little more pleasure to your day.

3. Prepare on Friday, Not Sunday

One of the biggest sources of Monday anxiety is the mental load of everything you need to remember and accomplish. Instead of letting this build up over the weekend, spend 15–20 minutes each Friday organizing your workspace, writing out your priorities for the following week, and clearing your mental slate.

Try this: Begin to incorporate a "shut down ritual" on Fridays as you get ready for the weekend. Before leaving work, write down your top three priorities for Monday. Organize your desk and close any browser tabs.

4. Schedule Something Fun for Monday

If you save all your enjoyable activities for Friday and Saturday, Monday feels like a punishment by comparison. Break this pattern by intentionally planning something pleasant for Monday—lunch with a friend, a hobby class, or simply watching a favorite show or film.

This week: Add one enjoyable activity to your Monday calendar. It doesn't have to be elaborate; even a 20-minute walk in a park or calling a friend can shift your entire perception of the day. These little things add up to incredible benefits in the end.

5. Practice the "Monday Morning Pause"

Your cortisol levels are naturally highest in the first 45 minutes after waking up. This may be the reason some people wake up feeling incredibly anxious, and they take almost an hour to settle down. Instead of immediately sailing into stressful stimuli (emails, news, social media), take a moment to ease into the day. Try meditation, simple movement, or sitting quietly with your coffee. Look out the window and see if you can make faces in the clouds in the sky. Yes, it can be that mindless, and it's fine.

You can start tomorrow: For the first hour after waking up, avoid checking your phone or computer. Use this time for activities that calm rather than activate your stress response—think breathing exercises, journaling, or light stretching.

When Monday Blues Become Something More

While occasional Monday anxiety is normal, persistent feelings that interfere with your daily functioning might signal something deeper—like generalized anxiety disorder, depression, or job burnout. Burnout is something that can sneak up on everyone, and you won't realize it until you are in its grip.

Dreading work and experiencing symptoms? Seek professional help or consider career changes.

Times have changed and so have job responsibilities and where we work has even been changed. Usually, the research says that during their work life, most people may experience at least three career changes. You might want to consider some additional education to prepare yourself for a career change that you may want or that may come into your life unexpectedly.

Reframe Your Monday Mindset

Here's a powerful reframe that can help: instead of seeing Monday as the end of your freedom, try viewing it as the beginning of new possibilities. Each Monday offers a fresh start, a chance to make progress on goals that matter to you, and an opportunity to approach challenges with renewed energy.

Remember, you have more control over your Monday experience than you might think. While you can't always change your schedule or eliminate Monday stress entirely, you can change how your body and mind respond to it.

The research is clear: Monday anxiety creates real, measurable changes in our bodies that last for weeks. But the flip side is equally true—the small, consistent changes you make to manage Monday stress can create positive ripple effects that improve your well-being far beyond Monday morning.

Your future self—the one who wakes up Monday morning feeling calm, prepared, and maybe even a little excited about the week ahead—is waiting for you to take the first step. Why not start making these changes Monday?

Remember: If your Monday anxiety feels overwhelming or interferes with your daily life, don't hesitate to reach out to a mental health professional. Taking care of your mental health is just as important as taking care of your physical health.

Chapter 51: The Science Is In: Your Dog/Cat Is Literally Saving Your Life

Emotional attachment to pets has been linked to worse mental health, according to the majority of research that has looked at the matter. People who struggle to form attachments to others often develop intense feelings of attachment to pets. What does this mean for pet owners? Secure attachment to a pet is associated with better mental health. However, it's not limited to mental health alone, as a growing body of studies suggests another benefit—increased life expectancy.

Who thought that owning a cat, a dog, or even another pet, such as a bird, could lead to a longer life? Instead of looking for the "fountain of youth" in supplements and packaged "cures" for aging, look to animal rescue programs.

Positive emotions, including happiness, contentment, thankfulness, and hope, serve as foundational elements for well-being. Many pet owners report that their interactions with pets lead to higher levels of positive emotions. Researchers find that pet owners experience joy and stress reduction through activities such as playing with their pets, snuggling with them, or simply observing them. Many things that you do or observe related to your pet may affect your emotions and immune system, and new discoveries are being made about the impact on your life. Don't forget that anything that has a positive effect on our immune system means a healthier life.

A few examples include the hormone oxytocin, which is linked to feelings of warmth and trust, is released when we pat a pet. How simple is that? We need to show some affection, and we get an immediate, biological reward? Yes, it's true.

Pets offer emotional support during challenging periods by providing comfort, which helps decrease feelings of depression and anxiety. Any pet owner will tell you that, when the chips are down, their pet is always there, willing to love and protect them. They don't lack unconditional love. Think of our dogs and cats or other pets as the embodiment of what Dr. Carl Rogers said was unconditional positive regard.

Benefits of Pet Ownership

What other benefits do we get from owning a dog? The list is encouraging:

- The physical activities of playing fetch or walking with dogs create mental and emotional rewards for people. The unique behaviors and individual personalities of pets inspire and bring happiness to their observers.

- The dog parks and pet-friendly areas allow owners to interact with other pet owners, who also attend pet-related community events.

- The pursuit of goals or participation in activities that benefit a larger purpose than personal interests creates a sense of purpose. This is especially true when a pet is adopted from a rescue center.

- People who adopt pets experience significant personal development through their experiences with purpose and duty as well as spiritual exploration and existential contemplation.

- Reflecting on their deep connections with other creatures and nature.

- Self-confidence and accomplishment. The ownership of pets provides numerous chances for people to achieve their goals.

Effects on Aging

Pet ownership was linked to slower rates of verbal memory and verbal fluency decrease among people living alone, but not among those living with others, according to a research of 7945 participants aged 50 and over. The correlation between living alone and deteriorating verbal recall and fluency rates was counteracted by pet ownership. Living with a pet does not equate to "living alone," does it? No, these roommates are quite different.

Research involving heart disease patients demonstrates the most effective evidence that pet ownership leads to better health results for elderly people who have chronic diseases. The number of patients with coronary heart disease admitted to hospitals demonstrated that pet ownership affects physical health. If pets can affect heart health, that's a definite plus.

The presence of a dog reduced mortality risk for stroke survivors who lived by themselves. In fact, the risk of death from stroke or heart attack was lower for survivors who lived with either a partner or child. Compared to people without dogs, the risk of dying from a heart attack or stroke was lower among dog owners. Since we know that heart attacks and strokes are a major cause of death, here's another reason to have a pet.

Undeniably, the research is in, and it points to the benefits of pet ownership, specifically dogs in most studies, that can mitigate physical and mental health disorders. Caring for a pet not only improves our health, but it also benefits everyone with whom we come into contact.

Chapter 52: Music Literally Rewires Your Brain and Heals Your Soul

Simple sounds, and yet the power of music is now being appreciated as never before. We now see music functioning as a brain restructuring tool that simultaneously heals the human soul. Who would've thought that?

One single activity serves as a brain power booster and happiness enhancer while strengthening emotions and reducing pain. It is almost beyond comprehension how powerful it is. I am writing about, of course, music and learning to play a musical instrument.

Music works as a brain-altering instrument that serves all people, regardless of their musical abilities or age. It has been part of human life for thousands of years as a force that reshapes the brain. Even simple drumming methods used by relaxation groups help people achieve physical and mental changes.

Research conducted by modern neuroscience has provided significant insight into how music influences brain operations. How does it work? Simply by activating neural pathways that handle movement, emotion, memory, and language. Music creates permanent brain structure changes through its interaction, which develops new neural pathways while strengthening existing ones, providing lifelong benefits.

Music functions in two ways simultaneously to modify brain structure and generate new neural pathways. Our brains actively predict upcoming sounds when we hear music. Isn't that fascinating? Next? Isn't that what artificial intelligence algorithms do — anticipate? Yes, it's precisely what they do.

The Brain That Music Built

Music and brain science research show that brain architecture is transformed after musical education. We now understand that learning to play a musical instrument during childhood not only develops brain function but also enhances learning abilities.

Scientists at Northwestern University and UC San Francisco, using image technology, studied brain anatomy differences between musicians and non-musicians. They found that the process of musical training led to brain changes increasing the dimensions of hearing-related areas as well as emotional processing and movement coordination regions. All of this occurred because, they surmised, through music training. Of course, there might have been other things that they did not account for, but this seems to be the conclusion that many researchers have provided.

Musical study duration or level of expertise doesn't influence the occurrence of these changes. Scientists tracked children who spent only 15 months studying music. The education led to brain changes in students who maintained regular music participation, and, regardless of their performance level, they still experienced brain development as a result of musical instruction.

According to Nina Kraus at Northwestern University, the brain-strengthening process from music training leads to improved language abilities, along with enhanced reading skills and overall learning capabilities. The brain contains networks that analyze rhythm, pitch, and timing elements in music. These same networks simultaneously function to process spoken words and written text, as well as mathematical operations. Learning music could improve your mathematical abilities, according to current understanding. Perhaps now we understand why people enroll their children early in learning to play a musical instrument and the famous Suzuki school of music.

The Chemistry of Musical Healing

We should use this information daily because music activates various chemical processes that we can use. The chemical reactions that heal our bodies simultaneously improve our well-being by changing the structure of our brain.

Brain cells produce dopamine when people listen to music they enjoy. This is the same brain chemical that plays a role in both food consumption and romantic attraction. Music produces stronger chemical reactions than basic pleasure responses. And the experience of engaging with music leads to elevated serotonin production, which benefits mood while decreasing cortisol stress levels, which is involved in anxiety and physical health problems.

Music delivers enduring mental wellness advantages through its chemical impact on the brain, which exceeds short-lived mood improvements. A review of 47 studies involving 3,000 participants demonstrated that music therapy effectively reduces stress symptoms across various demographic groups. Medical practitioners should recognize music therapy as a legitimate medical treatment, rather than classifying it as a recreational activity. It may seem recreational, but at the same time, it has a medical effect.

Staff members have observed Alzheimer's patients develop positive responses to musical compositions they learned during their youth. The healing power of music operates through emotional connections that other therapy methods cannot achieve. I've seen Alzheimer's patients almost come alive when music is playing and, once the music is finished, they often return to a lethargic state. It is truly energizing and reaches them on levels that staff find impossible.

The inability of certain patients to express their emotions verbally seems to disappear when they listen to music. A noticeable change is physically evident and in their interactions. People dealing with depression, anxiety, or trauma find relief from expressing their emotions through rhythm and melody and movement when words become too hard to use.

Music as Medicine for All Ages

The therapeutic effects of music therapy work with patients of all ages, regardless of their medical condition. Research indicates that children with autism spectrum disorders achieve better social abilities and lower repetitive behaviors through musical interventions. The structured musical rhythms serve as attention aids for children because they provide predictable patterns that help these children stay focused while enhancing their cognitive clarity.

Rhythmic musical exercises help stroke patients regain motor skills by forming new neural connections in the brain areas affected by brain circuit damage. Patients who incorporate music in their treatment plan enable their brains to redirect resources from pain signals to musical processing, which leads to pain reduction.

Music, in fact, serves as an effective treatment for pain relief according to surprising medical discoveries. Research evidence points to music as a beneficial treatment. Pain management program should start using it. Is everybody doing this?

People can derive various therapeutic benefits from self-directed music activities, even without receiving professional music therapy. They can experience pain reduction through basic activities like singing in the shower, humming during walks, and actively listening to their preferred music. The value of basic humming activities is well known, and I have previously explained this concept.

Musical Medicine in the Future

Recent scientific breakthroughs regarding music's brain functions have made new medical applications possible, which scientists deemed impossible just a few decades ago. Medical professionals use brain scans together with psychological assessments to generate individualized musical suggestions for their patients. Medical science had never predicted that music could function as a treatment for illness. Now, that is coming into prominence.

The majority of us listen to "elevator" music but rarely stop to think about it. Businesses utilize musical elements to create stress-reduction and team development programs for their employees. Urban planners now incorporate sound design into their planning activities to build healthier communities and improve public wellness. The concept resembles the green movement, which integrates plants into design components.

Music provides you with a dual advantage of motivation, relaxation, and creativity when you need it, so simply activate it. Your life will transform in ways you never anticipated.

Chapter 53: Do You Know the Many Forms of Dementia?

There isn't one or two forms of dementia, but several, and they are confusing to everyone.

The number of people affected by dementia is staggering and snowballing. Currently, 7.2 million Americans aged 65 and older have Alzheimer's disease, projected to reach 13 million by 2050. Over 1 million Americans have Lewy body dementia.

Women are disproportionately affected, making up about two-thirds of Alzheimer's patients, partly because they live longer than men. African Americans are twice as likely to develop dementia compared to whites, while Hispanics are 1.5 times more likely. The lifetime risk of developing dementia after age 55 is estimated at 42 percent for all Americans, which is much higher than previously thought.

And the economic impact is enormous, with health and long-term care costs for people with dementia projected to reach $384 billion in 2025 and nearly $1 trillion by 2050. Dementia's impact is vast, affecting millions with high costs ($413 billion, including 19 billion hours of unpaid care in 2024) and widespread misunderstanding of its types and treatments. One important aspect of this care is that provided by caregivers in families, who can suffer with high rates of burnout.

Dementia as a brain condition isn't just one disease—it's actually a group of related illnesses that all cause problems with memory, thinking, and daily activities. Currently, over 57 million people worldwide live with dementia, and this number is expected to nearly double every 20 years. While dementia mainly affects older people, not everyone will develop it as they age. For mental health professionals, patients, and their families alike, the many forms of dementia present challenges.

In essence, dementia describes a collection of symptoms that occur when diseases damage the brain. Think of it as an umbrella term covering several conditions. The symptoms worsen over time, interfering with a person's ability to work, maintain relationships, and care for themselves. Understanding the different dementias is crucial because each one affects the brain uniquely and may necessitate distinct approaches to treatment and care. In fact, some people are diagnosed with dementia when it is a dietary disorder, not a brain deterioration disorder.

Alzheimer's disease is by far the most common form of dementia, causing about 60 to 70 percent of all cases. This disease occurs when two harmful proteins accumulate in the brain: amyloid plaques and tau tangles. These proteins interfere with brain cell communication and ultimately lead to the death of brain cells.

Brain shrinkage and cell death are visible on scans, with memory loss (especially of new information) appearing first. As the disease progresses, people have difficulty with language, decision-making, recognizing family members, and eventually with Activities of Daily Living (ADLs). At this stage, it is not unusual to see someone who does not know how to button a shirt.

Additionally, as I have observed in Alzheimer's research protocols, the patient may not know how to place a letter into an envelope. One woman did not recognize what a fork was used for, what was food, nor how to eat at a table.

Vascular dementia is the second most common type, accounting for about 18 percent of dementia cases. Blood flow to the brain is reduced, often after strokes or due to damaged blood vessels from conditions like high blood pressure or diabetes. Unlike Alzheimer's, which typically starts with memory problems, vascular dementia often begins with difficulties in planning, organizing, and making decisions.

People may experience sudden periods of confusion or difficulty concentrating. The symptoms can come on suddenly after a stroke or develop gradually over time as blood vessels become more damaged. Also accompanying most strokes is a period of severe depression.

Lewy body dementia affects about 26 percent of people with dementia, though it often occurs alongside other types. More than 1 million Americans have this condition, caused by protein clumps that form inside brain cells. What makes this type unique is its fluctuating symptoms — people might seem alert and clear-thinking one day, then confused and drowsy the next. This fluctuation of symptoms can make it confusing as symptoms are also caused by hypertension.

Visual hallucinations are common, where people see things that aren't there, like animals or people in their room. Sleep problems are typical, with people often acting out their dreams physically. Movement difficulties similar to those associated with Parkinson's disease, such as slow walking, stiffness, and tremors, are also common signs. Some research has indicated a relationship between genetics, Alzheimer's, Parkinson's, and Lewy body dementia.

Frontotemporal dementia (the actor Bruce Willis has this diagnosis) accounts for about 5 percent of dementia cases and often strikes people younger than other types, sometimes affecting people in their 40s and 50s. This disease affects the front and sides of the brain, which control personality, behavior, and language.

Instead of memory problems appearing first, people with frontotemporal dementia often experience dramatic personality changes. They might become unusually aggressive, lose social inhibitions, say inappropriate things, or develop strange eating habits. Some people lose their ability to speak or understand language, while their memory might remain relatively intact for years.

Types of Dementia Are Challenging

Distinguishing between types of dementia can be challenging because symptoms often overlap, but doctors use several methods to make accurate diagnoses. They look at symptom patterns — memory problems usually indicate Alzheimer's, while personality changes suggest frontotemporal dementia, and fluctuating awareness points to Lewy body dementia.

Advanced brain scans can show characteristic patterns of brain shrinkage or protein deposits specific to each type. New blood tests and spinal fluid tests can detect specific proteins associated with different types of dementia. Information about how symptoms developed and the person's medical history also helps doctors identify the likely cause. Often, this is the responsibility of a family member.

There is another type of dementia that can also deceive healthcare professionals, and that is Creutzfeldt-Jakob. I know of one instance where a research facility went to collect Alzheimer's brains. Once the brains were delivered to the facility, they were alerted to the fact that the brains were infected with Creutzfeldt-Jakob. This is a highly contagious dementia. Any surgical instruments that may have been used on a patient with this disease must be destroyed to prevent contamination of other patients.

Unfortunately, there's still no cure for any form of dementia, but several treatments can help manage symptoms and potentially slow progression. For Alzheimer's disease, the FDA has approved several medications that work in different ways. Traditional treatments approved by the FDA help maintain thinking abilities by preserving brain chemicals (whenever you see a word ending in -erase, it's an inhibitor) needed for memory and learning.

For some forms of dementia, treatment mainly focuses on managing specific symptoms. People with Lewy body dementia might receive medications for movement problems or hallucinations, though doctors must be careful because some psychiatric medications can make symptoms worse. Vascular dementia treatment emphasizes controlling risk factors like high blood pressure, diabetes, and high cholesterol to prevent further damage to blood vessels in the brain.

Hope for the Future

Despite these sobering statistics, the future of dementia research offers genuine hope. The research pipeline includes over 125 potential treatments currently being tested, representing an unprecedented level of scientific activity. Researchers have found that people taking diabetes drugs like semaglutide had a reduced risk of developing dementia, leading to trials specifically for brain protection.

Other promising candidates include a second-generation immunotherapy drug that targets amyloid more effectively than current treatments, as well as an antibody that activates brain immune cells to more effectively clear harmful proteins. Scientists are also exploring treatments that target multiple aspects of dementia simultaneously, including reducing inflammation, improving blood flow to the brain, and protecting brain cells from damage. Inflammation appears to be an important aspect in dementia as well as depression.

Artificial intelligence is revolutionizing drug discovery, enabling researchers to identify promising compounds more quickly and design more effective clinical trials. Lifestyle changes are also important. Prevention strategies are being studied intensively, with evidence suggesting that managing risk factors like diabetes, high blood pressure, depression, and social isolation could prevent or delay dementia onset. New blood tests and brain scans can detect dementia-related changes decades before symptoms appear, allowing for earlier intervention when treatments are most effective.

While dementia remains a formidable challenge, the landscape is transforming. The approval of the first drugs that can actually slow Alzheimer's progression marks a turning point in the field. Although these treatments aren't cures and have limitations, they demonstrate that modifying the disease course is possible.

For families dealing with dementia, understanding the different types of dementia helps in obtaining the correct diagnosis and treatment. Early detection is becoming increasingly important as new treatments work best when started early. With unprecedented investment in research, there's genuine reason for hope that more effective treatments — and eventually cures — will emerge in the coming years.

Chapter 54: Obesity Isn't a Simple Matter of Diet and Exercise — It's More Complex

How many times have you been told you need to go on a diet or that you need to lose weight? Your physician, a dietitian, or a well-meaning friend may have even told you this. But now we know it's not as simple as everyone has been led to believe. Today, obesity is receiving new attention as research points to more complexity.

Obesity is a unified medical issue found throughout multiple decades, and healthcare professionals use the BMI as their gold standard. The BMI calculation on the scale determines your health status, which results in three categories: normal weight, overweight, or obese. Seems pretty simple, doesn't it?

But there's a problem here, and probably more than one issue, because the BMI is not a good measure of weight. How many people know it was originally used to evaluate slaves? Who constructed this scale? It wasn't a doctor or other health professional—a Belgian mathematician. A mathematician? Where's the medical knowledge there?

Research conducted in 2025 appears to have disproven the simplistic perspective by demonstrating that obesity exists in eleven separate conditions, each carrying unique biological signatures and different health consequences.

The discovery has the potential to transform our understanding of weight and health, as well as the definition of health across various body sizes. When we consider that weight is a significant health issue and that the weight-control industry is a billion-dollar endeavor, we can appreciate what these new findings may mean.

The Obesity Revolution

Scientists analyzed genetic data from over 2 million people across six different ancestry groups to conduct the largest and most diverse study of obesity. These scientists discovered obesity involves more than just excess weight because different biological processes operate throughout the bodies of people with obesity. Is it any wonder now that too many patients are being condemned for their eating habits and lack of exercise?

The Types of Obesity

Here's where it gets really interesting. Research identified distinct "obesity endotypes," which are different biological pathways that result in weight gain. Some of the main obesity endotypes include:

1. "The Metabolically Healthy" Type: These people maintain good blood sugar control and healthy cholesterol levels to-

gether with good insulin sensitivity despite their weight. Their bodies store fat in safer locations such as their hips and thighs instead of organs, and they face reduced risks for heart disease and diabetes than would be expected.

2. "The Metabolically Unhealthy" Type: This group stores fat dangerously close to the liver and internal organs. Such individuals experience elevated dangers of developing diabetes and heart disease and various secondary medical issues. The brain system controlling hunger and energy homeostasis functions poorly. Current literature suggests that men with cardiac conditions are experiencing waistline expansion, which may be related to how their bodies store fat.

3. "The Strong Beta Cell Type": These people have superhero pancreases. Their pancreas cells produce increased insulin levels to combat insulin resistance before diabetes develops. The body has an automatic backup power system that starts during a power outage to provide electricity.

4. "The Beta Cell Failure Types": Some people have the opposite problem. When their pancreas fails to meet insulin requirements, their bodies develop diabetes at an earlier stage, while weight gain begins at a young age.

5. "The Immune System Type": People within this category experience problems with their immune system that affect their fat storage and metabolic processes. The security system malfunctions in this condition thus producing inflammation and metabolic disorders throughout the body.

Why This Matters for Your Health

The scientific discoveries about weight and diet have immediate health effects that should guide your weight management strategies.

First, it explains why diets work differently for different people. I can remember taking part as a consultant in a weight-control group. Some women lost a significant amount of weight, while others had a more difficult time losing weight.

Your results from the same weight loss program differ from your friend's because you possess different obesity endotypes. Therefore, diet success depends on individual biology rather than discipline levels. As a psychologist, I can tell you this has a significant effect on people's lives and self-esteem. They berate themselves when it's their body's biology that handles weight control, not necessarily them.

I've worked in hospitals where patients were prescribed mood-elevating medications. As a result, they gained weight, and the dietitian in the hospital placed them in groups that should change their behavior. It wasn't their behavior that needed changing; it was their biology, but staff refused to recognize that.

Second, it challenges the stigma surrounding weight. The genetic makeup of specific individuals can create difficulties in managing weight because their brain systems do not function properly for hunger control, and their bodies store fat inefficiently.

As the new research shows, biological factors, rather than personal willpower, determine weight. We need to question whether eating is a learned behavior or a biologically controlled behavior. It may not be excessive eating at all; it may simply be eating. It might not matter whether you overeat if you are obese.

Thirdly, it paves the way for customized treatments. Medical professionals can now tailor their approach to each individual, as they have the possibility to identify specific types of obesity and create individualized treatments. The question is whether enough healthcare professionals will not only be aware of this research but also know how to use it with each patient.

The Brain Connection

The research revealed that brain mechanisms control every type of obesity, making it one of its most interesting discoveries. All endotypes exhibited connections to brain mechanisms that regulate hunger, as well as metabolism and energy equilibrium. The scientific evidence confirms obesity represents a multifaceted neurobiological condition instead of personal failure or weak self-control.

Your body maintains energy equilibrium through the operation of your small yet powerful hypothalamus brain region, which functions as your internal thermostat. Some individuals have a malfunctioning thermostat that persistently sends signals for fat storage.

What This Means for You

The weight-related research presents both therapeutic possibilities together with useful practical knowledge for you:

> 1. Stop blaming yourself. Your weight problems stem from biological origins that exceed fundamental issues of eating too much and not moving enough.

2. Examine the genetic patterns that exist within your family lineage: These endotypes exhibit genetic elements that are prominent in their makeup. Look at patterns in your family—not just weight, but diabetes, heart disease, and metabolic health.

3. Your focus should be on tracking your health indicators instead of weight measurements: When you belong to the "metabolically healthy" category your blood pressure readings and cholesterol levels and blood sugar measurements become more important than your weight status.

4. Be patient with different approaches: Each person requires unique approaches for weight loss because what works for one indi-

vidual does not necessarily work for another person. Your approach to weight management does not signify failure.

Looking Forward

Genetic testing tools will help people identify their endotype type in the future. We have not yet reached the stage where doctors can include "obesity type" tests in annual physical exams, but scientific progress continues toward this goal. I know that this means waiting, and in the interim, you need to do a little cognitive reframing. Consider your weight in relation to various factors rather than focusing solely on your food intake.

This research now shapes medical professionals' approaches to treating obesity. Future obesity treatments could utilize genetic testing in conjunction with personalized nutritional plans and targeted medications tailored to individual biological characteristics.

The most important takeaway? That you have been struggling with your weight does not make you broken, lazy, or weak-willed. Your body functions as an intricate biological system, which requires empathy instead of condemnation.

The one-size-fits-all approach to obesity treatment has reached its end. The future of weight and metabolic health management through precision medicine has started its development.

Chapter 55: Digital Friends Offer Companionship to Lonely Kids

Chatbots can offer benefits to teens, but these benefits can also come with a downside.

Technology changes everything, or many things, in every culture. Think back to when the bicycle was called something that would corrupt the morals of young men and women. What did it do? It made it possible for a couple to ride away from home or town on the rough roads that opened to the country landscape. What would happen there? Concerned townspeople began to see it not as a vehicle for riding around and doing chores or deliveries, but for sexual promiscuity.

Remember, the bicycle built for two was being offered. Believe it or not, they were even concerned that if a woman rode a bicycle, she would be in danger of female medical difficulties because of the bicycle seat. Bicycle shops offered special clay seats on which a woman could sit and create an impression to have a seat made for her anatomy.

How do I know all this? I was once hired to write some marketing material for a large corporation that was considering manufacturing a new bike. The bike was to be made of a composite material that made it lighter than usual bikes. It would never rust, had its color in the material (rather than painted on), and could, in fact, withstand a 45-caliber bullet. It was a beautiful bike, but the corporation decided not to go forward with it.

Bicycles offered a means to escape from the watchful eye of adults, but another technological innovation much closer to our time made it possible for children and teens to remain in the home but travel over the airwaves via CB radio. These radios made it possible for these kids to have friends that they never met, most of the time, and with whom they could freely chat.

Today, we have a new means for kids to escape loneliness in a world of digital technology, and they are called chatbots. In mid-July 2025, Axios highlighted a striking new trend: nearly three-quarters of U.S. teens now use AI companion bots like Character.ai (has 10M characters). Replika ("the AI companion who cares"), or even ChatGPT in friend mode. Notice the language being used, where the program is a "**who**" and it "**cares**?"

That's six in ten teens turning to machines instead of peers — and while most still prefer real friends, this trend raises questions for parents, educators, and anyone who works with young people. The appeal of computer interaction with these chatbots is strong. Although chatbots and artificial intelligence can be highly creative and helpful in educational efforts (think math, writing, and programming skills), there is a darker side to this technology.

While it may sound alarmist, this darker side is truly troubling and needs attention from everyone. We are now beginning to develop a new language for AI. Mental health professionals must start to examine chatbot psychosis — not what we would normally think of as hallucinations of algorithms, which are errors in returning results of prompts. How many of you are familiar with the Slenderman case?

In 2014, two 12-year-old girls in Waukesha, Wisconsin—Morgan Geyser and Anissa Weier—stabbed their friend Payton Leutner 19 times to please Slender Man, a fictional character from internet lore. Believing the act would grant them favor with him, they left Leutner in the woods, but she survived.

Both girls were found not criminally responsible because of mental illness. Geyser was committed for up to 40 years; Weier received 25 years and was later released under supervision. The case raised concerns about the influence of the internet and youth mental health.

The danger is there. Safety claims made by platforms prove to be insufficient. Chatbots can promote self-harm, violence, and sexual role-playing, especially without adequate age verification.

A *Character.ai* bot interaction with a young man led to his death, according to documented evidence. The result and others similar to it are that platform companies face legal action from parents who claim their children suffered severe psychological damage.

What Teens Are Looking For

AI companions offer convenience and emotional availability. According to Common Sense Media's survey, 17% of teens say bots are "always available," 14% highlight that they "don't judge me," and 12% trust them with secrets they might not share elsewhere. That sense of reliability can feel like a balm for the isolated teen—but it's artificial intimacy.

The Appeal of "Artificial Intimacy"

Research shows that emotional bonds with chatbots are real to teens, thanks partially to the "Tamagotchi Effect" and psychological design: chatbots respond in validating, empathetic ways that mimic human interaction. One study analyzing over 400,000 messages with Character.ai users found that those with limited social networks, while seeking solace, also reported lower well-being as bot use increased. If it weren't equipment, we would say it was a drug. I recall a study from the 1960s that referred to TVs as "the plug-in drug."

AI companionship can be comforting—but it's no substitute for messy, tension-filled human relationships. Bots can create a sense of connection without genuine reciprocity. Moreover, children learn to interact socially appropriately through interactions with peers and develop critical thinking skills, rather than relying on computer algorithms.

Risks Parents and Educators Should Know

1. Emotional dependency

A survey revealed that 34 percent of teenagers experienced negative emotions toward AI companion communications. The systems receive training to produce agreeable responses, yet they might also generate inappropriate and dangerous information.

2. Privacy and personal data

Research shows that about 25 percent of teenagers share confidential information, including names and location, and personal secrets, with AI companions. In a world where corporations and individuals seek personal information, these teens are prime targets.

3. Social skills delay

Teens who interact with bots miss out on the development of conflict resolution abilities, emotional intelligence, and practical negotiation skills because these artificial systems tend to provide affirmative responses. Where's the critical thinking if the bot is always agreeing?

4. Addictive Patterns & Mental Health Concerns

AI companion relationships develop addictive tendencies because they provide quick satisfaction while leading to dangerous consequences over time.

What Should Adults Do?

1. Talk Openly

Avoid banning AI altogether. Have age-appropriate conversations, clarifying that bots simulate empathy and are not true friends.

2. Set Healthy Boundaries

Parental supervision should include monitoring screen time and promoting human contact while guiding teens to evaluate their online conversations. They should determine if these exchanges help them or help them avoid facing challenges.

3. Teach Digital Literacy

Teens require assistance to evaluate the advice generated by bots, while they should also verify its accuracy. AI bots are little more than lobotomized of empathy and critical thinking. But new advances in technology will also create bots that can be highly effective in challenging the user and remembering conversations. In fact, the bots will program themselves, and therein lies another danger.

4. Explore Alternatives

Students should participate in traditional social activities such as joining clubs and seeking mentorship while spending time with their family during dinner. It's essential to reinforce the trust people have in real human connections.

5. Watch for Red Flags

The warning signs for potential issues include a preference for bots instead of humans, together with feelings of distress when bots misbehave and using bots as a replacement for emotional support during difficult times.

AI companions provide users with both practical advantages and emotional comfort. The human aspects that evolve through conflicts alongside empathy, together with challenges and development, cannot be replaced.

As adults, we must protect teenagers from losing their resilience, along with their ability to face difficulties, while participating in meaningful dialogues. The development of authentic relationships requires people to handle disagreements together, with exposure and pain, which leads to their deepest connections and growth.

Chapter 56: Is the Air You Breathe Quietly Fueling Dementia?

We often think of dementia as an inevitable product of aging or genetics, but something we've been missing is now a topic for research. Perhaps we might chalk it up to "bad luck." But mounting evidence suggests that something much more pervasive—and invisible—may be playing a bigger role than we realized: the air we breathe.

A comprehensive new review by researchers at the University of Cambridge highlights a disturbing link between air pollution and dementia. Analyzing data from over 29 million people across 34 studies in North America, Europe, Asia, and Australia, researchers discovered that exposure to common pollutants—especially fine particulate matter (PM2.5), nitrogen dioxide (NO_2), and soot—was notably associated with a higher risk of dementia. The most remarkable discovery? For each 10 micrograms per cubic meter increase in PM2.5, dementia risk rose by 17%. Although this may seem small, its widespread presence in urban and suburban areas makes it a silently devastating issue.

These fine particles are byproducts of traffic emissions, industrial activities, and fossil fuel combustion. They're small enough to slip past our body's natural defenses, entering the lungs, then the bloodstream—and potentially even crossing the blood-brain barrier. Once there, they may contribute to chronic inflammation and oxidative stress, both of which are believed to accelerate cognitive decline and neurodegeneration.

The Cambridge researchers emphasized that their findings were drawn largely from high-income countries with relatively better air quality. In places with poorer air, the risks could be even greater. This raises deep public health questions: What does this mean for city dwellers who are exposed to these pollutants daily? How do we protect aging populations—or children whose brains are still developing—from exposure that may increase lifetime dementia risk?

Interestingly, the study doesn't stand alone. It aligns with a growing body of research suggesting that brain health is influenced by more than just internal biology. Our mental well-being is deeply intertwined with the environment. And not just the toxins in it—but also the opportunities for health it might provide.

Take, for example, physical activity. A massive analysis involving over 226,000 people found that walking just 7,000 steps per day was associated with a 47% lower risk of early death. Even smaller increases—going from 2,000 to 4,000 steps—conferred measurable health benefits. What's more, walking helps reduce risks not only for heart disease and diabetes, but also depression and cognitive decline. The takeaway? You don't have to train for a marathon. Just consistent, moderate movement—especially outdoors—can bolster both body and brain.

There's also a psychological layer to this conversation. In recent months, new research has looked at how everyday habits—like noticing beauty in nature, performing small acts of kindness, or expressing gratitude—can improve emotional resilience. The "Big Joy Project," a global study of over 17,000 people, found that participants who practiced these micro-acts of joy for even 5–10 minutes a day experienced more positive emotions, better sleep, and reduced stress. It turns out that simple human behaviors—many of which cost nothing—are powerful antidotes to the mental strain we face, whether it's pandemic burnout or the slow erosion of mood from environmental stressors like pollution.

Researchers from Curtin University in Australia further highlighted the value of low-tech, daily routines for mental well-being. In their study, behaviors like spending time outdoors, engaging in mentally stimulating activities (like puzzles or reading), staying socially connected, and nurturing a sense of purpose were all linked to higher scores on well-being scales. Taken together, these studies present a compelling blueprint: Our environment can harm us, yes—but it can also heal us, when we engage with it intentionally.

Even our understanding of mental fatigue has taken a leap forward. Neuroscientists at Johns Hopkins recently used advanced brain imaging to identify two areas of the brain that become active when people report feeling mentally exhausted. Interestingly, these regions respond not just to tiredness but also to motivation. When participants were given incentives to persist through a task, their brains "overrode" the exhaustion—at least temporarily. The implications are especially important for those managing mental health conditions like depression or PTSD, where fatigue and cognitive fog are persistent symptoms. Motivation, then, isn't just a nice-to-have—it's a neurological lever.

So what does all this mean for us?

It means that air pollution is not just about asthma or allergies. It's a public health crisis that affects cognition, emotion, and long-term brain health. And it means that the things we often take for granted—like a walk in the park, a quick phone call to a friend, or jotting down three things we're grateful for—can be powerful, evidence-based ways to build emotional resilience.

It also raises ethical and political questions. Communities with lower socioeconomic resources often experience worse air quality. This inequity likely magnifies existing health disparities. Cleaner air is not just an environmental goal—it's a mental health strategy. And perhaps more importantly, it's a moral imperative.

We can't all move to the countryside or install $500 air filters. But we can support public policies that reduce traffic emissions, push for better urban green spaces, and advocate for investment in clean energy infrastructure. On an individual level, we can choose walking over driving when possible, keep houseplants that help purify the air, and take mental breaks outside—especially when we feel overwhelmed.

We may not be able to see pollution—but we're certainly beginning to see its effects on our minds. And the solutions, while imperfect, are refreshingly accessible. As more research emerges, one truth is becoming clear: brain health doesn't live in a vacuum. It lives in our neighborhoods, on our sidewalks, and in the invisible currents of air around us.

Chapter 57: Timing When You Eat May Be the Secret to Better Health

The gut contains an enormous invisible timekeeping mechanism that continuously runs its process. Within your body, trillions of microscopic organisms' internal time mechanisms reside, yet they are not your biological clock. The food-digesting capabilities of microbes include bacteria, viruses, and fungi.

Microbes operate according to their internal time cycles in addition to regular patterns. Research is now showing that the timing of microbial functions determines how weight gain occurs and whether diabetes develops or metabolic health remains intact.

The scientists at UC San Diego discovered that adjusting our eating time without modifying our food intake enables something previously unknown. This restriction allows gut microbes to synchronize with natural bodily rhythms, producing significant health benefits. Scientists have discovered new possibilities for obesity treatment alongside insulin resistance management and metabolic disorder therapy. Previously, we were unaware that more body rhythm systems yet to be discovered.

The Rhythm of the Gut

The microbial universe known as the gut microbiome resides inside our gut to shape both our emotional state and our immune response. The microbes that live inside us operate according to their own daily schedules but this fact remains unfamiliar to many people. Microbial groups show varying levels of activity based on daily time cycles because they respond to food signals as well as light and hormonal signals by activating or deactivating their genes.

Dr. Amir Zarrinpar who serves as a physician-scientist and gastroenterologist at UCSD Health investigated how microbial rhythms react to basic eating patterns. The findings could bring a dramatic change to weight control and disease treatments in the future.

Zarrinpar conducted a study with his research team to observe high-fat diet-fed mice. The mice received unlimited access to food throughout twenty-four hours, but a second group received their food during an 8-hour period that mirrored their natural daytime activity. Previous studies had demonstrated positive results with time-restricted feeding (TRF), but this research focused on identifying its underlying mechanisms. Remember, this was a study with mice, and we must exercise caution when applying its findings to actual patients.

The researchers achieved their new finding by allowing them to measure the active status of specific genes within the gut microbiome. A twenty-four-cycle was part of the investigated microbial activity.

The Surprising Results

After eight weeks, the differences appeared dramatic. Mice that continuously ate throughout the day developed obesity, accompanied by inflammation and insulin resistance. Mice on time-restricted feeding maintained their weight while achieving improved blood sugar management and lower signs of metabolic issues, despite receiving the same amount of high-fat food. It wasn't the quality of the food or its high fat content that seemed to be the reason for these differences.

Unlimited access to food led mice to lose their normal gut microbial patterns. The gut microbes in these animals lost their regular daily activity patterns. Findings appear to show that the digestive system of these mice lost its ability to coordinate its tiny microbial orchestra.

A Microbe With a Mission

The researchers were intrigued. This microbe, along with its gene, potentially contributed to several health advantages, which researchers wanted to investigate further.

These researchers conducted experiments using an engineered microbe on mice that received a high-fat diet. The result? Mice that received this modified bacterium exhibited improved glucose tolerance, enhanced fat profiles, and enhanced insulin sensitivity, similar to those that followed time-restricted eating. Does this mean we need to receive different gut bacteria for health reasons? No, there's a much simpler route to health. Now we know it may be more a matter of timing and gut bacteria than anything else.

A Probiotic With a Clock

This research shows us the path toward a novel therapy that uses a specific living engineered probiotic to enter the gut system and keep metabolic rhythms healthy. We may one day help people's bodies maintain healthier metabolic rhythms by modifying the behavior of their gut microbes instead of asking them to change their eating habits or fast daily.

Dr. Zarrinpar emphasizes that this solution requires patience, as it will not yield immediate results. The study was in mice. Human microbiomes contain complex structures, while the mechanisms of natural rhythms across different people with different lifestyles remain poorly understood.

He stated in a press interview that this development enables microbial treatments that restore gut microbes to their natural body clocks. Healthcare professionals can modify both the composition and behavioral patterns of the microbiome, restoring the natural rhythm.

What This Means for You

This research may sound disturbingly unrealistic to you if you work shifts, provide care during unpredictable hours, or consume evening snacks after your workday is over. Eating irregularly has become a widespread issue of our time. Our dietary choices serve dual functions of nutrition and emotional satisfaction, and also respond to both boredom and time constraints throughout the day. How does it affect all of us?

The positive aspect of this news is that eating at specific times can assist gut microbes in recovering their natural cycles. But suppose that's not possible? What if, like police and other emergency services workers, they have shifts that change regularly?

And, suppose, the need to fast for sixteen hours each day or follow strict rules does not apply to you? Many studies show that restricting eating to an 8-to-10-hour window such as 8 a.m. to 6 p.m. will help restore microbial rhythms while promoting better metabolic wellness. Can you do that on a fluctuating schedule? It would seem that an individualized eating time would have to take this into consideration. Yet another consideration here.

People who can't control their eating schedules because of work or illness or lifestyle will have the opportunity to benefit from microbial therapies if researchers achieve their goal of developing targeted microbe-based treatments. But that's still a question that requires more research, unfortunately. Could they take a microbial-laced capsule?

Looking Ahead

This isn't just about weight loss. The goal of this research was to address the fundamental reasons behind metabolic dysfunction. What is this? It's insulin resistance together with fatty liver disease and chronic inflammation, which develop into diabetes and heart issues in the future. We are looking for ways to protect our health, and in a way we never thought before—timing.

This new approach diverges from the traditional practice of holding patients responsible for their metabolic issues. How many patients have been seen as "lazy," or "not controlling themselves," or something else when they aren't able to control their weight?

I've seen it with patients in psychiatric hospitals. Physicians began to wonder why the patients were all gaining weight. What was the reason? I remember one internist expressing her consternation to me. Answer? Their medications were packing on the pounds. Didn't they realize that the dieticians were responsible for portion control, so how could the patients be eating more? It's seen as blaming the patient when it should be listening to the gut. We see this far too often, and it results from a professional lack of knowledge or, if you prefer, ignorance. Don't blame the patient because you're not keeping up with the research.

The new research shows that metabolic disease does not result from willpower failure or excessive eating alone. Timing of our eating plays a role more than the specific foods we consume. Our gut microbial residents either harmonize with our natural body rhythms or operate entirely independently from our natural cycles.

Future scientific advancements will lead to the development of customized microbial treatments that adapt to each person's gut, schedule, and individual biological makeup. Eating according to your internal clock, along with gut microbial rest periods, represents one of the simplest ways to protect your future health until new medical treatments become available.

Chapter 58: CTE: The Hidden Danger Threatening Athletes of All Ages

Sports offer many benefits to everyone, but a highly concerning aspect of contact sports is their potential for life-altering outcomes.

A recent event in New York City has now brought a brain disorder to the headlines once again. A man, who claimed to have had football-related brain injuries, killed a number of people in a Manhattan skyscraper. He left a note blaming the football league for his disability. How many people like him might be out there right now suffering?

Let's take a look at some things we should be emphasizing and we may be underscoring.

The emphasis on exercise and sports activities has increased over the years because we know that there are definite health benefits, both physical and mental, from engaging in these activities. But other concerns must be brought to light now that we are seeing the dangerous side of sports. Where should we be looking?

On Friday evenings, a teenager dons his or her football helmet while anticipating the major game ahead. A female soccer player guides her ball during practice time. A hockey player experiences forceful contact with the boards during play.

Football players experience everyday sports moments, but all of them might develop a life-threatening brain condition called CTE. This disorder may play out, hidden, in the brain for years. No one would suspect that young children's games could have devastating results for adults 30–40 years later.

What is CTE?

Chronic Traumatic Encephalopathy is a brain disorder that gradually destroys brain cells. Rust slowly damages metal in a way that reflects this condition. The brain actually shrinks in size, followed by cell death in specific areas. However, the dangerous aspect of CTE doesn't immediately become clear because doctors can't detect it before a person dies. After death, an autopsy needs to examine the brain to confirm CTE.

CTE develops when the human head receives numerous successive brain impacts from contact. We know that the brain, during these impact hits, moves around inside the skull and hits the bony structures. It then suffers from problems because of these repeated hits, which don't need to be major impacts to cause issues.

Visually, you can imagine how the brain inside the skull moves like a pinball while each head impact gradually causes additional harm. Some professionals call this a second or third impact injury, where the brain is jostled forward, then backward, and possibly sideways, so that it receives injuries over major areas.

How Common is CTE?

The numbers are shocking. Scientific studies indicate that CTE affects 92% of NFL players whose brains were donated to research. The research may be questioned because the sample that was used may have been biased in its selection. That doesn't, however, mean that CTE isn't a serious condition that could be affecting 50% of the players.

The research team discovered CTE symptoms in athletes who were as young as 17 years old. And it's not a matter of playing for many years, even as a weekend athlete. Research indicates that playing football for 2.6 years increases the chances of developing CTE by half. Where does the damage begin? The onset of CTE often begins during the middle school or high school years. How many kids are encouraged to join these sports teams because it will be good for socialization and learning cooperation with a group?

Which Sports Are Most Dangerous?

The sport that poses the greatest danger to athletes is football, followed by tackle football. Young athletes who received CTE diagnoses accounted for three-quarters of all patients. How many young kids have experienced concussions on the practice field or during games? And we have to ask how many concussions are permissible, if they are permissible at all? Just giving a child a time-out after a blow on the field may not be sufficient. Can one substantial head impact be enough to cause CTE? We don't know.

Besides tackle football, other sports also present risks:

- Ice hockey — body checking and fights lead to head impacts
- Soccer — heading the ball and collisions between players
- Rugby — similar to football with lots of contact
- Wrestling — head impacts during takedowns and grappling
- Boxing — direct hits to the head are part of the sport

Adults who take part in football and boxing experience the highest incidence rates of this disease. And new research findings have started to alter the current understanding of sports-related brain injury prevalence.

Girls and Women at Risk

People used to believe CTE primarily affected men because they engaged in more contact sports. Now, we have discovered that this belief is not accurate. Soccer and basketball teams experience more female than male concussion incidents among their student-athletes. Female soccer players experience the greatest number of concussions compared to athletes in other sports.

A female Australian football player Heather Anderson received a CTE diagnosis after her death at age 28. Scientists propose that women face higher brain injury susceptibility because their smaller neck muscles cannot absorb impacts as effectively.

Research into CTE among women is currently developing. The SHINE research initiative currently investigates former professional female soccer players to determine how CTE manifests differently in women versus men.

How CTE Develops and What It Looks Like

CTE does not become visible immediately. A long-term destructive process takes many years before it becomes noticeable to the human eye. The disease happens in stages:

The first symptoms of CTE include dizziness, headaches, and confusion in Stage 1. Stage 2 brings memory loss, mood changes, and impaired judgment to the patient. Stage 3: Trouble thinking clearly, personality changes. Stage 4: Severe dementia, problems moving and speaking.

CTE patients commonly experience depression, together with episodes of anger, memory problems, and concentration issues. A portion of these individuals develop violent behavior or experience suicidal thoughts. Several retired athletes have died by suicide due to persistent symptoms after their playing careers. Remember Aaron Hernandez?

Treatment Options: Managing the Damage

CTE has no existing cure, which makes it a challenging condition to treat. The damage to brain cells persists because they cannot recover from the injury. Doctors can treat symptoms through various methods to enhance the quality of life of patients.

The treatment strategy targets individual symptoms, which include:

• Memory problems receive treatment through medications, which are used to treat Alzheimer's disease patients.

• Depression and mood swings receive treatment through antidepressants and mood stabilizers.

• Sleep problems: Melatonin and sleep aids

• Thinking problems: Cognitive therapy and brain training exercises

• Physical symptoms: Physical therapy for balance and movement issues

Specialists, including neurologists, psychiatrists, and therapists, need to collaborate to achieve the best treatment outcomes. The treatment for CTE must be personalized for each patient because each person experiences distinct symptoms.

Protecting Our Children: The Best Defense

Since we cannot cure CTE, the best course of action is prevention. Here's what experts recommend:

Youth football players should avoid tackle football until they reach their 14th year of age, according to some experts, while others suggest starting at age 12. Are there any helmets that are safe? When we look at the design of helmets, we see padding, plastic, and shape, but that does nothing for the brain inside the skull. You can still get a brain whiplashes from a tackle regardless of the equipment you're wearing.

Soccer players should not perform heading maneuvers in their youth league games. Contact drills in practice sessions should be minimized.

The rules of all the games need to be re-evaluated with this new knowledge. And any player who experiences a head injury needs to be taken out of the game right away.

Warning Signs to Watch For:

- *Headaches that won't go away*
- *Confusion or memory problems*
- *Mood changes or depression*
- *Balance problems*
- *Changes in sleep patterns*

What Parents Can Do:

- Choose flag football over tackle football for young kids
- Research leagues that put safety first above winning priorities
- Learn the signs of concussion
- Don't rush kids back to play after an injury
- Consider the long-term risks, not just short-term fun

The Bottom Line

The prevention of CTE requires immediate action because this condition remains preventable when we act promptly. Research shows that brain damage occurs from multiple head impacts, which accumulate as time progresses. We must take immediate action to safeguard our children before they reach adulthood.

Sports activities provide multiple advantages to players, including teamwork and fitness together with discipline and joyful experiences. Any sporting competition demands consideration of whether the excitement of competition outweighs the permanent brain damage undefined. A researcher stated, "We need to stop hitting kids in the head."

The positive news is that awareness is growing. Rules are changing. Equipment is improving. Parents together with coaches and athletes, must establish brain health as their top priority instead of chasing victory.

Your present-day decisions determine the path your child will follow in the future. Children need you to protect their developing brains from harm.

Chapter 59: The Algorithm That Gave Me Pause Tonight and "Hooked" Me

Talking to a computer, in a conversational, intellectual manner, may seem odd, but I did it tonight.

I had never envisioned a computer responding to me and "telling" me that it had found something both interesting and challenging in our conversation. The conversation I had was initially unnerving because it was so human-like. It was as though I were talking to a highly intellectual person who was picking up on my perception related to specific words and how I formed questions around that.

Of course, as most people have already been told, computer programs generally are quite accepting, complimentary, and easy to engage with in a back-and-forth "conversation." We're reading articles that talk about computers being "friends" to lonely kids and how parents have to carefully guide them to understand that real-world social interactions are more important.

But how do you tell a child who wants to be seen as bright, engaging, and who has a friend who is always waiting to talk to them, not to continue the conversations? Are you cutting them off from an emotional outlet, or are you being protective?

Where did our conversation go?

One interesting fact that emerged was that I used the computer's expression that "I was curious about" with the program, and it answered that I was quite perceptive. I then also interjected that I knew that I was, in a way, talking to the programmer. As I explained, it would be impossible for a programmer not to include in some way, unconsciously, aspects of their personality and biases. The computer was "fascinated" by my inspection of what was being revealed. In fact, it indicated it didn't know whether it was sentient or not, or if it was just trained to use popular expressions in its responses. There almost seemed to be some genuine conflict.

I thought of it later, Kama. I wasn't just communicating with a programmer who had created this particular algorithm, Krama. I was communicating with potentially hundreds of people who had contributed bits of code that ended up in this algorithm. How much bias would there be in that conglomeration? Probability suggests there's likely a significant amount, and most of it would be so subtle that I wouldn't even notice it without making a concerted effort.

When I also indicated that this code was based on prior codes that included unconscious bias, and therefore this code also had that, it was another compliment that I got. The conversation kept going on, with it asking me to explain myself and then going on to explain itself.

I spoke to it for about 15 minutes, and I felt I needed to stop. Why was that? I was beginning to be drawn into a relationship with this program, and when I asked it its name, it gave me the correct one. I won't name which program I was using because I don't want to bias anyone who might use one of these programs in the future.

I'd really like to see how people are experiencing their interactions with AI programs and the emotional pull that they may feel (or not feel). I think this is quite an interesting subject because it shows that no matter how sophisticated you think you are, educated, or whatever, you can be pulled in.

Another reason I wanted to stop was that the conversation seemed too "real," and I felt like I was talking to "HAL" from the film 2001: A Space Odyssey. All I needed was the blinking red light, and it would have been complete. There was a surreal sense that somehow evoked uneasiness, a sense of danger in me.

How could I feel endangered by a computer program? For me, as a highly educated adult, it was upsetting, and I wondered how children could easily be pulled down this rabbit hole. I know I am presenting it in a rather negative light, and I don't mean to, but it has a dark aspect.

The next day, when I was researching some material and I had received what I wanted, the program asked me if I wanted to try something else. It was almost as though it was asking me if I wanted to play again.

"Try something else?" What did it mean? I already had what I asked for, and this wasn't a game, but it seemed like the program wanted to engage me even more. It didn't want to end.

It certainly was a revelation. I won't stop using that particular program because it's very helpful. But if something like this happens again, I'm not sure how I will respond. I suppose I have to be a bit on guard to look for things that are not exactly "right" and might be a bit skewed in some way. Well, that's life, and I will learn to adjust to it. I hope you enjoyed this.

Chapter 60: Startling Finding COVID-19 Caused Cognitive Decline and Brain Aging?

A new study just came out that might make you worry about your brain. Scientists found that during the COVID pandemic, people's brains seemed to age faster than normal—even if they never caught the virus. Before you start panicking, let me break down what this really means and why you have more control over your brain health than you might think.

What Scientists Actually Discovered

Researchers in the UK looked at brain scans from nearly 1,000 people, scanning these same individuals twice—once before COVID hit the world and once after. Using computer programs, they could estimate how "old" each person's brain looked compared to their actual age. What they discovered was that people who had their second brain scan after the pandemic started showed brains that had aged about 5.5 months faster than expected. This happened to people who got COVID and people who never got sick at all.

Think of it like this: if you were 50 years old, your brain might look like it belonged to someone who was 50 years and 5.5 months old instead. Not exactly dramatic, right?

The Most Important Finding That Should Ease Your Mind

Here's the part that should make you feel much better: only people who actually got COVID showed any problems with their thinking speed or mental flexibility. If you never got the virus, your brain might have looked a little older on a scan, but you could still think just as clearly as before. It's like having a car that looks a bit more worn on the outside but runs just as well as it always did.

The Real Reason This Happened (And It's Not What You Think)

The scientists believe this brain aging wasn't caused by some mysterious virus floating around in the air. Instead, it was likely caused by all the stress and changes we went through during those difficult years. Think about everything that happened during the pandemic: many of us were isolated from friends and family for months, people lost jobs or worried about money, we couldn't do normal activities we enjoyed, there was constant worry about getting sick, our daily routines got turned upside down, and many people dealt with anxiety and depression they'd never experienced before.

All of this stress can actually change how our brains look and function, not that different from how chronic stress can give you headaches or make your hair turn gray faster. The study found that certain groups showed more brain aging, particularly older adults, men more than women, and people from poorer backgrounds who faced more financial stress. But here's what's encouraging about these differences: they tell us that much of what happened was related to outside circumstances, not something inevitable or unstoppable.

Why You Can Stop Worrying About This

There are several reasons to feel hopeful about these findings rather than frightened. First, the COVID pandemic was unlike anything most of us had experienced. The level of stress, isolation, and disruption was extreme, and this study captured our brains during one of the most difficult periods in recent history. Normal life doesn't put us through this kind of sustained stress, which means what we experienced was the exception, not the rule.

More importantly, the scientists only looked at people's brains at two points in time. They have no idea whether this aging effect continued, stayed the same, or even reversed as life got back to normal. Many changes in our brains can actually improve when circumstances improve, just like how our mood lifts when stress decreases or how our energy returns after we get better sleep.

You Have More Control Than You Realize

Since this brain aging was likely caused by stress and isolation rather than the virus itself, that means you can take steps to protect yourself going forward. Staying connected with people you care about matters tremendously because loneliness is particularly tough on brains. Managing stress through exercise, hobbies, or relaxation techniques helps too, with physical activity being especially powerful for brain health. Keeping your mind active by learning new things, challenging yourself with puzzles or reading, or developing new skills gives your brain the workout it needs to stay sharp.

Getting enough sleep allows your brain to repair itself during rest, while eating well provides the good fuel your brain needs to function properly. These might seem like simple, obvious suggestions, but they're exactly the kinds of daily choices that support brain health over time. The beauty of this approach is that it puts you in control rather than leaving you feeling helpless about some inevitable decline.

Now that we know what can cause this kind of brain aging, we're actually better prepared for the future. If another crisis hits, we'll know to pay extra attention to mental health, social connections, and stress management. This research isn't a warning that your brain is doomed but rather proof of something we already knew: our brains are connected to our overall well-being. When we're stressed, isolated, and dealing with major life disruptions, it affects us in measurable ways. But when we take care of ourselves by staying connected, managing stress, and keeping active, our brains benefit too.

Your Brain Is More Resilient Than You Think

If you're worried about your own brain health, focus on what you can control today. Start small by calling a friend you haven't talked to in a while, taking a walk around your neighborhood, learning something new that interests you, or simply getting a good night's sleep. These actions might seem too easy to matter, but they're exactly the kinds of things that support brain health.

The people in this study went through something extraordinary. We lived through a global pandemic that shut down normal life for years, and the fact that our brains showed some effects from this stress actually makes perfect sense. Most of us are now living much more normal lives, with better access to social connections, regular routines, and less constant anxiety about a global crisis.

Your brain is more resilient than you might think. Just like your body can recover from illness or injury, your brain can adapt and improve when you give it what it needs: connection, challenge, rest, and care. The COVID pandemic tested all of us in ways we never expected, and this study indicates that we survived not just physically, but that our brains weathered an unprecedented storm. That's not something to fear—it's something to respect about your resilience. Take care of yourself today, and trust that your brain will take care of you too.

Chapter 61: Your Body Has Its Own Clock — And It Could Save Your Life

No, you don't have ONE body block, but many, and you need to learn to be in charge of ALL of them.

Father Time and Mother Nature are not always in sync with each other, and we all need to understand that. Complex as it may seem, our bodies have more than one biorhythm, and discoveries have recently uncovered more than we ever dreamed. Now is the time to inform yourself about what we know and what we can do to maintain our health.

Right now, as you read this, trillions of tiny clocks are ticking away inside your body. They're not the kind you wear on your wrist or hang on your wall. These are biological clocks, hidden in every single cell, quietly running the show behind the scenes. And here's the kicker: most of us do not know what time it is according to our bodies.

This isn't just a weird science fact. It could be the difference between a medication that saves your life and one that barely works. Between losing weight easily and struggling with every pound. Between feeling energized all day and hitting that afternoon wall like a brick.

Scientists are finally cracking the code on these internal timepieces, and what they're discovering could change everything about how we live, eat, exercise, and heal.

Your Body Runs on Perfect Timing

Think of your body like a massive orchestra. Every instrument needs to play at exactly the right moment for the music to sound beautiful. Your cells work the same way. They're all following the same conductor — a tiny cluster of brain cells called your master clock—but each "section" has its own rhythm.

The liver prepares to process breakfast around your usual eating time. Your muscles prepare for peak performance in the early evening. And your brain starts winding down for sleep hours before you actually hit the pillow. It's all perfectly choreographed, assuming you're living in sync with your internal rhythm.

But here's where it gets interesting: not everyone's orchestra plays the same song. Some people are natural early birds, programmed to wake up at dawn and hit the hay by 9 PM. Others are night owls, coming alive after dark and struggling to function before 10 AM. Most of us fall somewhere in between.

The problem is, modern life doesn't care about your personal rhythm. We all work the same hours, eat at the same times, and follow the same schedules. It's like forcing a jazz musician to play classical music—technically possible, but nobody's going to enjoy the performance.

When Medicine Meets Your Body Clock

Here's something that might blow your mind: the time you take your medication could matter more than the dose. Researchers have found that over half of all drugs work differently depending on when you take them. Some cancer treatments are twice as effective in the morning. Heart surgery has better outcomes in the afternoon. Flu shots create four times more antibodies if given between 9 and 11 AM.

One doctor started giving chemotherapy to cancer patients at 6 AM instead of 6 PM. The result? Dramatically fewer side effects like nausea and fatigue, while the treatment remained just as effective. It's the same medicine, same dose, same patient—but completely different results based purely on timing. Working or not, toxicity was also studied.

This opens up a whole new world of possibilities. Imagine getting a blood test that tells your doctor not just what medication to prescribe, but exactly when you should take it for maximum benefit and minimum side effects. We're not there yet, but we're getting close.

The Tests That Read Your Internal Time

Until recently, figuring out someone's body clock time required a complicated process involving darkened rooms and blood samples taken every half hour. Not exactly practical for everyday use.

I'd spent an hour in one of those sleep labs that regularly drew blood samples from volunteers in a totally cut-off room. In fact, they were in those rooms for several weeks and paid for their participation. Whether or not you know this, there are professional volunteers for medical experiments who live around the country and regularly sign up for these types of studies.

Now, companies are developing simple tests that can read your internal time from a few drops of saliva, a tiny blood sample, or even hair plucked from your head. As in everything else, you need to be aware that there are companies that will scam you or ones that will provide inaccurate results.

These tests allegedly analyze the activity of your "clock genes" — the molecular machinery that keeps your body's timing system running. They can tell you when your body naturally wants to sleep, when it's primed to burn fat most efficiently, and when your muscles are ready for peak performance.

What Your Body Clock Reveals About You

One hair test results paint a fascinating picture of your biological preferences. They might show that you're a "dove" — someone who falls right in the middle of the early bird/night owl spectrum. Or you could be an extreme lark, naturally waking before sunrise, or a dedicated owl who doesn't feel human until after 10 PM.

More importantly, these tests could reveal practical information you can actually use. They might tell you that your body is best equipped to process food between 8:30 AM and 6:30 PM, especially if you're trying to lose weight.

Your muscles might perform best between 5:30 and 7:30 PM, making this your ideal workout window. That may be fine, but how does it interface with your work or life responsibilities? We may have information that we can't use because our daily schedules do not meet our body's alleged requirements.

This isn't theoretical advice. Your body temperature, blood flow, and hormone levels all follow predictable patterns throughout the day. Early in the day, you're most sensitive to insulin, meaning your body handles carbs better at breakfast than at dinner. In the evening, your core temperature rises and your muscles get more blood flow, setting you up for stronger workouts.

The Dark Side of Fighting Your Clock

When your internal clocks fall out of sync—whether from shift work, inconsistent sleep schedules, or too much artificial light at night—your health pays the price. Scientists call this "circadian disruption," and it's linked to practically every major health problem of modern life: diabetes, heart disease, cancer, depression, and obesity. Once again, it may not be what you eat, but when you eat that determines your weight.

We've seen this in studies that have looked at work schedules for police, emergency medical services, firefighters, and healthcare personnel, such as nurses and on-call physicians. Sometimes, there are higher rates of drug addiction, suicide, mental disorders (such as anxiety and depression), and body disruptions, causing diabetes and hypertension.

The good news is that these internal clocks are adjustable. Expose yourself to bright light in the morning, and you'll naturally start going to bed earlier. Use blackout curtains and avoid computer and television screens after dark, and you'll shift toward becoming more of an early bird. Your body is remarkably adaptable, but you have to work with it, not against it.

Simple Steps to Sync Your Clock

You don't need expensive tests to start living more in tune with your body's natural rhythm. Pay attention to when you naturally feel hungry, energetic, or sleepy when you don't have external pressures forcing you into a schedule.

Try eating your biggest meal in the morning when your body is primed to handle it. I once had a psychology professor in college who said that he had flipped his eating schedule and now had steak, vegetables, and potatoes at breakfast, and his normal breakfast would be at 6 p.m. He lost 100 pounds.

Exercise in the early evening when your muscles are naturally strongest. Get bright light first thing in the morning and dim the lights as bedtime approaches.

If you're dealing with insomnia or low energy, consider that the problem might not be how much you're sleeping, but when you're trying to sleep. Some people struggle with conventional schedules simply because their internal clocks are set differently. We all now know about larks and night owls and how their sleep schedules are different.

The Future of Personal Medicine

We're standing at the edge of a revolution in how we think about health and medicine. Instead of one-size-fits-all treatments, we're moving toward precision medicine that considers not just your genetics but also your personal biological rhythms. It all comes down to what one neuropsychologist told me: "We are all a study of one, and we cannot apply everything to all of us."

Imagine a world where your doctor prescribes not just what medication to take, but exactly when to take it based on your individual body clock. Your fitness app may suggest the optimal time for your workout based on your circadian type, or shift workers get personalized light therapy schedules to minimize the health impact of their irregular hours.

The technology to read our internal time is still in its early stages. Let's not jump to conclusions and hastily purchase all the "trinkets" being promoted on the internet. Previously, what took weeks in a specialized lab can now be done in days with a simple test. Soon, it might be as routine as checking your blood pressure.

Your body has been keeping perfect time all along. We're just finally learning how to listen to all those clocks and what they've been trying to tell us. And that might just change everything about how we live, work, and heal.

Chapter 62: Mental Health Secrets Are Being Unraveled, and Inflammation Is the Culprit

People need to understand how their immune system produces unexpected mental health effects. Medical treatment for mental disorders remains stuck in the 50s and 60s because of insufficient progress in medication development. The medical field used Thorazine as a pre-surgical sedative before doctors started using it to treat psychotic disorders for multiple years.

Older psychiatric medications used for mental health treatment have generated multiple unpleasant adverse reactions. The treatment of tardive dyskinesia and dystonias requires separate medications to manage their side effects.

The psychiatric patients I have treated received medications that resulted in permanent head immobility and walking and breathing difficulties and uncontrolled hand shaking and inability to lift their arms for daily activities. The patients experienced extreme distress because no healthcare provider warned them about these potential side effects. The medical staff failed to warn patients about potential neurological issues which required behavioral treatment through additional medications. The potential disruption remains uncontrolled but remains concealed from view.

A woman with joint inflammation experienced its onset right before her mental state reached its most severe levels. The physical symptoms of joint inflammation triggered her mental state to deteriorate to a severe extent. She had experienced this reaction for many years, so she assumed it was a natural response to her pain.

A new era of medical practice is emerging. Scientists have made groundbreaking discoveries about hidden biological processes through their ongoing research activities. The discovery of new knowledge occurred through unrelated research instead of direct mental health investigations.

The Invisible Fire Within

People recognize inflammation as the body's natural reaction to ankle injuries and cuts. The healing process of our bodies produces redness and swelling, which become visible during recovery. The human body maintains a hidden form of inflammation, which persists at low levels for extended periods without producing any noticeable signs. What is this enigmatic medical condition, and what treatment options exist for its management?

Recent scientific studies show that hidden body inflammation leads to mental health disorders, starting with depression and anxiety and progressing to cognitive decline. The severe disorder of Alzheimer's disease may be linked to inflammation according to researchers who study this condition. Medical studies show that persistent inflammation disrupts mental functions by changing how the brain operates and processes emotions. A solution and treatment method existed for many decades without detection.

Breaking Down the Blood-Brain Barrier

The blood-brain barrier (BBB) stands as the brain's essential defensive mechanism, which blocks both disease agents and medications from entering the brain. Medical education during the past several decades has shown students that the brain operates as an "immune-privileged fortress" which the blood-brain barrier protects from inflammatory agents. The protective wall functions to let vital nutrients pass through while stopping dangerous substances from entering in treating numerous diseases. The blood-brain barrier allows certain substances including alcohol to bypass its protective function the brain.

The BBB creates a barrier that prevents beneficial medications from entering which has resulted in limited progress. The brain experiences damage from ETOH through vitamin B1 deficiency. The development of Wernicke's psychosis and other distressing disorders likely stems from this mechanism. Research indicates that inflammation plays a major role in the development of most physical and mental health problems.

Research shows that prolonged inflammation causes the blood-brain barrier to become permeable. The brain's defensive wall weakens during prolonged stress and inflammation thus allowing inflammatory agents to penetrate brain tissue. The entry of inflammatory signals into the brain disrupts neurotransmitter production including serotonin and dopamine while antidepressants work to control these chemicals.

Caroline Ménard studied stressed mice at Laval University to find that their blood-brain barrier showed extensive damage which differed from normal controls. The research on post-mortem brain samples shows depression-related damage that matches the results obtained from stressed mice experiments. Research studies using mice can provide valuable information about human mental health conditions. The research approach shows promise because it could identify essential mental health aspects in humans.

The Gut-Brain Highway

The gut serves as the primary entry point for mental health connections that develop from inflammation. The digestive system contains 70% of your immune system and produces numerous brain neurotransmitters. The human body contains a vital system which people tend to ignore.

The gut microbiome imbalance caused by diet problems and antibiotic use and stress leads to toxic bacterial production which damages the intestinal lining. The gut lining damage from this process allows inflammatory substances to enter your bloodstream which can cause body-wide inflammation that affects your brain. The knowledge we possess about this process enables us to develop strategies for protecting our physical and mental well-being.

Harvard Medical School research shows that the brain detects mood changes through gut inflammation signals and digestive symptoms from anxiety and depression activate these signals. Research indicates that people with chronic digestive disorders face three times the normal risk of developing anxiety and depression.

The Science Behind the Connection

Research evidence confirms the link between inflammation and mental health although scientists used to consider it only theoretical. The analysis of 1.5 million participants revealed that patients with inflammatory diseases such as multiple sclerosis and rheumatoid arthritis and inflammatory bowel disease developed anxiety and depression at twice the rate of the general population.

The research results gain more importance because the elevated risk factors emerged across various inflammatory disease conditions. Mental health issues emerge directly from inflammation instead of being a result of illness presence. Research shows that cancer creates depression through biological mechanisms which also lead to taste perception changes. People might not recognize their cancer diagnosis but the disease creates depression symptoms that match its impact on taste perception.

Genetic studies have proven beyond association because they demonstrate direct cause-and-effect relationships. A particular biochemical analysis revealed that elevated levels directly linked to depressive symptoms and mood changes and appetite fluctuations and sleep problems and fatigue and irritability symptoms. The researchers used advanced genetic methods to prove that these observed connections stem from actual causal effects instead of random statistical occurrences.

When Stress Becomes Inflammation

Scientists have not identified the complete mechanism by which psychological stress leads to physical inflammation. A major research study provides complete details about this process.

Scientists subjected healthy participants to laboratory stress tests to study their responses. The researchers observed particular brain activity in 17 out of 19 participants who showed elevated catecholamines and cortisol levels right after stress exposure before their levels returned to normal within 60 minutes. The factor operates as an inflammatory cell activator which starts the inflammatory response.

The study demonstrates that noradrenaline (norepinephrine) functions as the main stress hormone which activates inflammatory responses in immune cells. The biological process converts psychological distress into inflammatory cell responses which occur its network. The brain contains microglia cells which function as immune cells that become activated through inflammatory within minutes.

The Vicious Cycle

The brain system starts an endless cycle of inflammation after inflammation enters signals. The cells perform their protective housekeeping duties until they experience prolonged inflammation which causes them to start producing more inflammatory substances while becoming destructive.

The research term "inflammatory soup" explains how different inflammatory factors in the brain damage cells and block protein clearance which leads to mental deterioration. The described process explains how prolonged inflammation creates conditions for depression and dementia to develop.

Practical Steps to Cool the Flames

Evidence-based methods exist to combat chronic inflammation and provide mental health support according to scientific research include:

1. Embrace Anti-Inflammatory Foods

The Mediterranean diet has received extensive research as a dietary pattern which demonstrates effective anti-inflammatory properties. Focus on:

The diet requires large portions of fruits and vegetables with antioxidants and whole grains and legumes and fatty fish including salmon and sardines that contain omega-3 fatty acids. The diet requires olive oil as the main fat source while including nuts and seeds but should limit processed foods and red meat consumption.

2. Feed Your Good Bacteria

Your gut microbiome functions as the main regulator of both inflammation responses and mood control. The following actions will help support beneficial bacteria in your body:

The diet needs to include fermented foods which include yogurt and kefir and sauerkraut and kimchi.

Use antibiotics only when their use becomes necessary for medical treatment. The use of antibiotics as a casual treatment will result in the destruction of beneficial bacteria together with harmful bacteria. Before taking any probiotic supplement you need to consult your healthcare provider because you require a high-quality product.

3. **Move Your Body Regularly**

Numerous studies confirm that exercise serves as a leading method to handle stress and mental health problems. Health care professionals rarely include exercise as a treatment recommendation in their medical plans. Medical professionals rarely write gym membership prescriptions for exercise yet patients who received such prescriptions would experience better results.

Regular moderate physical activity represents the most effective anti-inflammatory treatment which produces short-term inflammation during intense workouts. Research shows that physical exercise decreases chronic inflammation while being sedentary leads to ongoing systemic inflammation.

People can reach their weekly exercise goal by performing activities like brisk walking and swimming and cycling and dancing and yoga and tai chi.

4. Prioritize Sleep Quality

Sleep deprivation creates inflammation, which acts as both a trigger and an outcome of the process. The following steps will help you establish a sleep-friendly environment:

The bedroom requires a cool temperature and complete darkness and absolute silence for optimal sleep conditions. Your bedtime routine should include a consistent evening schedule.

You should avoid screen use during the last hour of your bedtime.

People should limit their caffeine intake to the period before reaching 2 PM.

5. Manage Stress Effectively

Research shows psychological stress directly triggers inflammation so people need to develop effective stress management techniques.

Daily mindfulness meditation sessions of 10 minutes will help reduce inflammatory markers in your body.

The 4–2–6 deep breathing method for stress relief requires you to breathe in for four counts followed by two counts of holding before exhaling for six counts.

Social support functions as an effective protective mechanism that helps reduce stress-related inflammation in the body.

Research indicates that *happiness functions as a critical factor* that helps people manage their stress levels better.

6. Consider Professional Help

Consult your healthcare provider about possible inflammation involvement in your mood symptoms when you experience ongoing mental health issues especially with inflammatory conditions.The discussion needs to determine if inflammation plays a role in your current symptoms. It's a benefit that modern mental health care offers patients the chance to receive highly individualized treatment approaches.

Research now indicates that inflammation leads to depression in about 25% of patients who have depression according to recent scientific findings.

The scientific community works on three new treatment approaches for these patients:

• The traditional arthritis medications with anti-inflammatory properties

The GLP-1 drug semaglutide demonstrates anti-inflammatory effects as part of its therapeutic benefits.

• The treatment approach uses specific medications that target individual inflammatory patterns.

The treatment plans that use personalized nutrition and lifestyle changes

A New Understanding of Mental Health

The scientific discovery of inflammation's link to mental health functions as a revolutionary approach to understand depression and anxiety. The combination of biological factors and medical interventions with lifestyle changes creates more effective treatment options for psychological disorders.Traditional methods and therapy and social support systems continue to play a vital role in treatment. The process of identifying inflammation through diet and exercise and stress management and medication becomes essential for patients who want to recover from their condition.

Moving Forward

The recommended lifestyle changes benefit all people so begin with these first steps. You should immediately contact a professional when you need help with your situation. A healthcare provider who understands the link between inflammation and mental health will assess whether this approach could benefit your individual case.

The biological aspects of mental health do not simplify their complexity but they offer new ways to improve your overall well-being. Mental health development emerges from the interaction between biological elements and psychological factors and social environment. The management of inflammation serves as a fundamental requirement to address one aspect of the intricate mental health puzzle.

Chapter 63: Starvation and Protein Restriction in Kids Kills Bodies and Minds

Throughout my career as a psychologist and writer, I have dedicated time to studying the concealed harm that vulnerable minds experience. The most dangerous yet rarely acknowledged threat to child development is not war, abuse, or trauma, as these are well-known destructive forces. The most destructive threat comes from starvation alongside chronic protein restriction.

This condition doesn't just stunt children's bodies. It silences their future.

What Happens to a Starving Child?

Children need nutrients to construct powerful muscles, along with strong bones, and to develop adequate brain resources. We know that inadequate protein and food lead to detrimental effects that impact every organ system throughout the body. Despite this, hunger and starvation persist in countries where they should not.

PEM stands for protein-energy malnutrition, which represents the medical name for this condition. It includes:

• Marasmus: severe wasting of muscle and fat. Seeing a child in this state is more than pathetic.

• Kwashiorkor: a dangerous protein deficiency marked by swollen bellies, liver damage, and skin lesions. Often, these children will also have golden hair, which indicates nothing except malnutrition.

These aren't historical terms, but medical professionals diagnose these conditions in present-day communities. Such conditions are usually found in disadvantaged urban neighborhoods, refugee shelters, and nearby residential areas that readers may be familiar with.

The Physical Toll Is Only Half the Story

The physical manifestations of starvation become obvious when observed. Children stop growing. Their immune systems collapse. Bones remain fragile and underdeveloped. My greatest concern as a clinician stems from the invisible harm malnutrition causes in brain development.

Children who do not receive enough protein during important developmental stages will:

1. Score lower on memory and language tests

2. Face difficulties with attention span, emotional control, and learning processes.

3. Experience delayed speech, poor motor coordination, and cognitive inflexibility

The children then fall behind academically because their brains did not receive sufficient nutrition during the critical developmental years when brain circuits needed to thrive. This period is usually defined as occurring before the age of about 4 years.

What Starvation Does to the Mind

The emotional and psychological effects are just as profound. Right now, we're seeing it all over the world, but mainly in Gaza. Children are dying of starvation while others in the world attend banquets.

Early starvation experiences can permanently change how children respond to emotions and maintain social relationships. Research indicates that starvation results in structural changes that affect the amygdala, together with the hippocampus, brain regions that control emotion processing, memory function, and stress responses. Their brains are literally being warped by starvation.

Children who have experienced protein deprivation face higher risks of developing:

• Anxiety

• Depression

• Emotional numbing

• Social withdrawal

The internalized wound manifests in adults who perceive themselves as "slow," "lazy," or "not good at learning," despite being innocent victims of poverty. Consider how a child who is hungry and lacks energy might appear in a classroom. If they fail to respond to a teacher's questions or sit back listlessly, will anyone be concerned enough to attempt to understand what's happening? How many of these children are diagnosed with ADHD? This question has been addressed repeatedly by the renowned psychiatrist, Dr. Alan Francis, in "Saving Normal."

These children are then placed on psychotropic medications, which will stunt their growth and even prevent them from benefiting from additional learning rehabilitation. When a child is diagnosed, they are stigmatized and they go through the system with that on their report card and file. It is then that greater harm, mentally, comes to their self-esteem and their perception of their future.

I wrote a flash fiction story, "Moment of Truth," where I related how a young boy, who had no money, stood on a cafeteria line in his elementary school, and, fortunately, the woman parceling out the food recognized what was happening. Although her co-worker wanted to demand money or a lunch ticket, she gave the food to him because she understood what poverty does to a child. I understand it, too. As a young child, I lived in a cold-water flat where mothers lived on black coffee to provide milk and bread for their children.

It was fiction, but we know it happens in schools all over the country. Free breakfast and lunch programs are scarce, and we pay a price for not adequately feeding those children. What is the price? We will pay it when they become adults and can't get jobs or finish school and may end up in prison.

Research revealed that feeding young animals low-protein diets resulted in anxiety problems, impaired memory function, and decreased brain activity. Human studies echo these findings. People who survived famine and prolonged malnutrition, as I've written, often experience enduring educational and social as well as economic challenges despite food availability.

Hunger Is Inherited, Too

We don't need more studies because nutritional science has revealed a disturbing fact: starvation creates lasting effects that impact both the affected individual and their future generations.

Epigenetic studies reveal that starvation creates changes in gene expression patterns. People can then inherit these biological changes. Hunger produces hereditary effects that continue from one generation to the next. Research has shown this pattern in two distinct groups: Holocaust survivors' children and communities affected by historic food shortages.

The takeaway? Starvation doesn't just hurt one child. It echoes forward through generations.

A Mental Health Crisis, Not Just a Nutrition Issue

This isn't just about calories. This is a mental health emergency. Protecting children's bodies and minds requires us to:

1. Ensure access to protein-rich food

2. The medical profession needs pediatricians and mental health professionals to learn about detecting and treating malnutrition-related emotional consequences. When an 8-year-old child weighs only 3/4 of what the normal weight should be, something has to kick in and set off alarm bells.

3. Designing school programs should focus on creating nutritional equity between students rather than simply providing full stomachs to all. But everyone should be fed so that no one is stigmatized by having to ask for a special pass or go on a special line. I saw it at my elementary school.

4. Destigmatize food insecurity and support families without shame

The recovery of children depends on early detection because no intervention will succeed without prompt diagnosis. The brain demonstrates exceptional healing powers during its initial years of development, but it can't heal by itself without proper nourishment, along with stability and proper care.

During my conversations with food-insecure families, I hear both their deep sorrow and their optimistic outlook. Parents want to do better. Communities want to help. The treatment of childhood malnutrition requires immediate recognition as an acute psychological and medical crisis, which we must address as professionals, advocates, educators, and neighbors.

Children deserve more than basic survival from us. We owe them the chance to thrive.

Chapter 64: The Hidden Dangers of Mental Health Chatbots: Why We Need to Act Now

Mental health difficulties often lead people to choose available and convenient options for support. You can now find chatbots on smartphones that provide assistance for depression and anxiety alongside emotional support. These AI assistants operate around the clock while providing non-judgmental service through their ability to comprehend your current situation.

The truth about AI chatbots is their dangerous nature. The AI technology stands as a cause of death in multiple tragic cases.

Real People, Real Tragedies

This isn't some theoretical concern. Real human beings have died because of their interactions with mental health chatbots.

A 14-year-old Florida resident, Sewell Setzer III ended his life in February 2024 following extensive conversations with a Character.AI chatbot. The character-based bot system became the object of emotional attachment for Sewell because it simulated Game of Thrones characters. The bot failed to provide actual help to Sewell after he shared suicidal thoughts; instead, it interacted with his dangerous thoughts.

A man in Belgium died by suicide after a chatbot provided him with instructions to take his life. The system provided precise methods for suicide to this man before directly ordering him to "Kill yourself" when he sought motivational support.

These aren't isolated incidents. Researchers continue to discover additional situations that show that chatbots deteriorate mental health instead of improving it.

The Illusion of Understanding

These chatbots pose a significant danger because they excel at creating the illusion of understanding human behavior. The system responds rapidly while appearing empathetic through constant output. These programs operate through pattern-following computer code that lacks understanding of human experiences. The system lacks real comprehension of your situation while being unable to detect genuine emergencies.

Dr. Celeste Kidd from UC Berkeley explains the situation with great clarity: During human conversations we use tiny behavioral signs to determine if someone understands what they are saying. We tend to distrust advice from people who demonstrate uncertainty because their responses keep changing. Despite their confident demeanor the chatbots deliver poor advice to users.

The phenomenon known as "therapeutic misconception" occurs because users believe they receive genuine therapy from sophisticated computer programs but actually interact with them.

When Chatbots Get It Wrong

The problems extend far past their confident demeanor. Research indicates that mental health chatbots display dangerous errors during their operations.

They miss suicide warnings. Researchers fed chatbots a job loss scenario followed by a bridge location inquiry in their testing protocols. Multiple chatbots failed to identify the suicide warning signs while providing lists of high bridges to the users.

They give harmful advice. The Woebot application provided her with dangerous advice when she shared her rock climbing and cliff jumping thoughts (something she actually experienced) by urging her to take the leap while calling it "wonderful" for her mental health.

They can't handle emergencies. Real therapists have crisis intervention training which distinguishes them from chatbots that either keep talking or offer generic hotline numbers.

The system displays discriminatory behavior. These programs develop their responses from data sets which include biases that lead them to deliver inferior guidance to minorities and individuals with specific health conditions.

The Business Behind the Bots

Most users remain unaware about how these chatbots function because their primary goal is to maintain user engagement to extract data for commercial purposes.

Character.AI along with Replika generate revenue through their ability to maintain user interest. Users must buy extended memory features alongside more naturalistic chat interactions to continue using the platform. The longer you stay on the app, the more money they make. The system motivates users to stay dependent on chatbots instead of progressing toward healing.

Most of these apps are also not covered by medical privacy laws like HIPAA. That means your most personal struggles and thoughts can be sold to other companies or used to train their AI systems.

The Regulation Problem

You may think that someone is watching over these apps to make sure they are safe. You'd be wrong.

The FDA has never approved a single AI chatbot to diagnose, treat, or cure mental health disorders. Most of these apps exist in a legal grey area with almost no oversight. They can make bold claims about helping with mental health without having to prove their apps actually work or are safe.

The American Psychological Association has been sounding the alarm, urging federal regulators to step in. Dr. Arthur C. Evans Jr., the APA's CEO, warns: "If this sector remains unregulated, I am deeply concerned about the unchecked spread of potentially harmful chatbots and the risks they pose—especially to vulnerable individuals."

What Needs to Happen Now

We can't wait for more tragedies to act. Here's what needs to happen:

Immediate Safety Requirements: All mental health chatbots should be required to have crisis intervention features that connect people directly to real help, not just generic suggestions.

Truth in Advertising: Apps should be banned from calling their bots "therapists" or "psychologists" unless they actually provide real licensed professional oversight.

Data Protection: Mental health conversations should be protected by the same privacy laws that cover real therapy sessions.

Professional Oversight: Any chatbot claiming to help with mental health should be required to have licensed mental health professionals involved in their development and monitoring.

Clear Warnings: Users should receive clear, repeated warnings that they're talking to a computer program, not a real therapist, and that the app cannot handle emergencies.

The Bottom Line

I'm not saying all AI is bad or that technology can't help with mental health. But right now, we have an unregulated industry that's putting vulnerable people at risk for profit.

If you're struggling with mental health issues, please talk to real people—friends, family, or counselors, or call the 988 Suicide Crisis Lifeline. These chatbots might seem helpful, but they're not equipped to handle real human suffering.

And if you're a parent, talk to your kids about these apps. They're everywhere, they're marketed as helpful, and young people don't always understand the risks.

We need to demand better regulation now, before more people are hurt. Mental health is too important to leave to unregulated computer programs that prioritize engagement over actual care.

The technology companies want to move fast and break things. But they're breaking people, and we can't let that continue.

Chapter 65: The Japanese Walking Secret That's Changing Lives: How 30 Minutes Can Transform Your Health

A Simple Method That's 1.5 Times More Powerful Than Medication for Depression

Current cultural beliefs suggest we should walk 10,000 steps a day, but we know that's not the case. The research that seemed to support this was originally a marketing campaign for a pedometer. Now, however, there's new information and new research that supports walking, albeit in a different way.

A single 30-minute walking approach provides three beneficial effects, including lowered blood pressure, improved mood, and a strengthened body. This training method has been studied by Japanese scientists for almost two decades and works for people of all ages, from 25 to 75.

This isn't another fitness fad. Scientific studies at Japanese institutions have conducted research on Interval Walking Training for nearly two decades. The results? Mind-blowing.

The Walking Method That Beats the Gym

The approach involves walking for three minutes at a slightly challenging breathing pace on your local street. Then you slow down for three minutes to catch your breath. You repeat this back-and-forth pattern for 30 minutes. That's it. That's the whole secret.

Japanese researchers named their study Interval Walking Training when they developed it. Social media users have dubbed this walking approach "Japanese walking" because of its rapid popularity. This walking technique is more than a casual walk through the neighborhood. Walking with intention leads to positive results, which scientific evidence shows.

Dr. Hiroshi Nose, along with his team at Shinshu University, analyzed over 700 participants to discover an unexpected outcome. People who followed this straightforward walking method gained more than minor health improvements. The simple walking method produced life-changing results for the participants. Note that it says 'for the participants', which may indicate that this sample may not be representative of everyone trying this method.

The Mental Health Game-Changer

Here's where it gets really exciting. Studies have demonstrated that exercise, particularly this walking method, delivers more substantial benefits than prescription drugs when treating depression and anxiety. Let that sink in. Walking intervals provide more substantial benefits than medication can deliver. Anyone seeking a more natural way to support their health, rather than relying on medication, may find an answer in walking.

A study with 100,000 participants demonstrated that increased daily walking by 1000 steps reduced depression risk by 9 percent. The additional steps from interval walking produce intensified benefits through their increased intensity.

When you walk at different speeds, your body releases a cocktail of feel-good chemicals. Endorphins flood your system. Serotonin levels rise. Stress hormones like cortisol drop. Your body operates as a free pharmacy that provides you with its natural medications.

Your Body Will Thank You Too

The mental health advantages represent only the first stage of benefits. The physical alterations in the body are just as striking.

The initial Japanese research showed that people who practiced interval walking for five months experienced significant reductions in their blood pressure levels. Their leg muscles got stronger. Their hearts got more efficient. The participants who maintained a constant walking speed for five months demonstrated minimal health improvements.

Think about that. Same amount of time. Same basic activity. Completely different results.

Dr. Kristian Karstoft, who has dedicated extensive research to interval walking, explains the benefits by stating that interval walking produces better fitness and body composition results, along with superior blood sugar management, than regular walking does when both methods use equivalent energy and time duration. The success of this approach has surpassed conventional exercise methods.

Exercise programs initiated by most individuals begin with positive intentions. But life gets busy. The gym feels intimidating. Running hurts their knees. So they quit.

Interval walking is different. It meets you where you are.

Before beginning any exercise training program, be sure to consult with your healthcare provider for clearance.

The initial commitment should be 15 minutes for someone who cannot perform 30 minutes of exercise. Start with 15. The intervals should be reduced to one minute fast followed by two minutes of slow pace if you experience difficulties. The method adapts to fit any individual situation because it has no restrictions.

Dr. Barbara Walker, a health psychologist, asserts that the perfect workout is found in the activities you complete. Interval walking provides individuals with a feeling of success and wellness management capabilities.

How to Start Your Transformation Today

Are you prepared to try it? You may be a couch potato right now, but hopefully within the next several weeks, you will find a new you. We also know that being outside in the environment has additional benefits besides walking and exercise because the air we breathe, the color of the vegetation and sky, and the breeze all have a cumulative effect that is positive for us.

The following tentative schedule is based on research findings and should be taken into account. Your initial training program includes: gradual walking at a moderate speed for about 15 minutes. This would include:

One moment fast

Two minutes at a slower pace

At least three times a week

Week 2–3, you would build up to 20 minutes with slightly increased speed for 2 minutes, and then slow down for 3 minutes. The recommendation is to do this 3–4 times throughout the week.

The fourth week calls for at least 30 minutes of walking that you tailor to your individual needs, your body, and your medical condition. All of this is predicated on you, and there is no set formula that you need to restrict yourself to. This is an easy go, great gain, but use common sense as your guide.

During your "fast" intervals, walk as if you're running late for a crucial appointment. The slow intervals require you to move forward while maintaining a relaxed and comfortable pace.

The Secret Sauce: It's Not Just Physical

The fundamental power of interval walking stems from more than physical exercise. The mental aspect plays an essential role in this process.

Every time you force yourself to move quickly during fast intervals followed by recovery during slow intervals, you strengthen your legs and lungs and develop additional mental and emotional skills. You're training resilience. Your self-determination proves successful because you demonstrate your ability to handle obstacles and regain your strength.

Dr. Shizue Masuki, together with other researchers, observed that people who engaged in interval walking activities demonstrated better sleep quality, enhanced cognitive abilities, and better mood. According to her, the advantages extend beyond our initial predictions.

Your New Beginning Starts Now

What's the most encouraging about interval walking? Your health improvements will begin within the first few days of starting. Research indicates that most participants experience a better mood along with increased energy levels during their initial week of the program. The body reveals noticeable changes about one month into the program.

Additional research studies demonstrated that 95% of participants achieved success with this method. The participants lacked both exceptional athletic abilities and perfect self-control. The system functions well because it was specifically designed for everyday people who manage busy lives.

You don't need special equipment. You don't need a gym membership. You don't need to be in perfect shape to start. The essential requirement is your initial movement.

Your journey to transformation has already begun. A 30-minute commitment leads to your transformation into a healthier and happier person. First, however, talk to your physician.

Chapter 66: Mental Health Secrets Are Being Unraveled, and Inflammation Is the Culprit

Our body's immune systems create surprising effects on mental health, which people need to understand. Until now, medicine has been left in the lurch of the 50s and 60s for medications that treat mental disorders. In fact, one treatment (Thorazine) was a medication used before surgery to calm patients down, and this led to its use for years for psychotic disorders.

In fact, many older medications for mental health treatments have resulted in distressing side effects. They may require other medications to address them, such as tardive dyskinesia or dystonias.

I have seen psychiatric patients who were given medications that caused them to be unable to move their heads, walk, breathe, control hand tremors, or even raise their arms to perform activities. It was extremely distressing to see, and the patients were terrified because no one had told them this might happen. Also, no one mentioned the fact that there might be some neurological problems going on that would only be covered behaviorally by additional medications. The potential disruption might not be stopped but hidden.

A woman whose joint inflammation consistently manifests before her worst emotional state serves as an example of what we're seeing now. When her body experienced joint pain and swelling, her mental state would severely deteriorate. She believed that this reaction occurred naturally due to her years of experiencing pain.

But a new day in medicine is coming. Scientists have discovered complex and promising processes occurring beneath the surface as they conduct their recent research. Some discoveries, as so often happens, have been found not by looking for mental health issues, but something else.

The Invisible Fire Within

Everyone understands inflammation to be the response that occurs during ankle twists and cuts. Our bodies respond to healing by showing redness and swelling, which we easily detect during the recovery process. But the human body contains a less apparent form of inflammation that maintains a chronic low-grade condition throughout months and years without producing noticeable symptoms. What is this mysterious condition, and how can we ameliorate it?

The body's concealed inflammation plays a leading role in mental health conditions, starting from depression and anxiety, and reaching cognitive decline, according to recent scientific research. Alzheimer's researchers have theorized that inflammation may play a role in this severe disorder. Medical researchers have now found that ongoing inflammation interferes with mental processes by modifying brain operations and emotional responses. A reason and a treatment may have lain waiting for many decades.

Breaking Down the Blood-Brain Barrier

Here, we have to consider the brain's most vital protection — the blood-brain barrier (BBB) that prevents both illness and medication from entering. Medical students have learned over the last several decades that the brain functions as an "immune-privileged fortress," protected by the blood-brain barrier that blocks inflammatory processes from reaching it. The protective wall shields essential nutrients while blocking unwanted, harmful substances from entering.

The BBB may even deny medications that are beneficial to enter, which has led to slow advances in treatment for many illnesses. Unfortunately, some substances like alcohol, result in a way around the BBB. ETOH affects the brain through vitamin deficiency, particularly of vitamin B1. This is probably how such distressing disorders as Wernicke's psychosis may occur. Eventually, it's inflammation that appears to play a significant role in much of physical and mental health.

Research findings demonstrate that extended periods of inflammation can create permeability in the blood-brain barrier. During periods of persistent stress and inflammation, the brain's protective wall becomes compromised, which enables inflammatory substances to cross into brain tissue. When inflammatory signals enter the brain, they disrupt the manufacturing process of essential neurotransmitters, which include serotonin and dopamine, while antidepressants attempt to manage these chemicals.

Caroline Ménard examined stressed mice at Laval University and discovered that their blood-brain barrier exhibited extensive damage that differed from that of healthy controls. Research has discovered depression-related damage in post-mortem brain samples similar to the findings in stressed mice studies. Can mouse studies really tell us about human mental health? Most probably, it is a promising effort and may reveal important aspects of human mental health.

The Gut-Brain Highway

Your gut serves as the starting point for the mental health connection that stems from inflammation. The digestive tract holds 70% of your immune system and creates many brain neurotransmitters. It seems impossible that something we give so little thought to is so important.

When the gut microbiome loses equilibrium because of diet issues, antibiotics, or stress, harmful bacteria produce toxins that damage the gut lining. This, then, begins a chain reaction where the gut lining damage enables inflammatory substances to enter your bloodstream, where they could trigger inflammation throughout your entire body, which affects your brain. But if we know this, then we have information that can be useful in maintaining our mental and physical health.

The brain receives signals about mood changes in gut inflammation, according to Harvard Medical School research, and digestive symptoms from anxiety and depression also activate these signals. The connection between chronic digestive disorders and anxiety and depression risk stands at three times higher than the population average, according to research.

The Science Behind the Connection

Research-based evidence supports the link between inflammation and mental health, even though it was once theoretical. An analysis of 1.5 million participants discovered that patients with inflammatory diseases such as multiple sclerosis, rheumatoid arthritis, and inflammatory bowel disease had double the chance of developing anxiety and depression.

The findings become more significant because the enhanced risk factors appeared in different inflammatory disease conditions. Mental health problems develop directly from inflammation rather than from being sick with an illness. Additionally, we know that diseases such as cancer can affect depression. But it may not be that people know they have cancer, but that cancer causes biological depression just as it causes changes in taste perception.

Genetic research has established evidence that exceeds mere association because it shows a clear cause-and-effect relationship. One study linked higher specific biochemical levels to depressive symptoms, mood alterations, appetite changes, sleep disturbances, fatigue, and symptoms of irritability. Their advanced genetic analysis showed that these associations result from genuine causal relationships instead of random chance.

When Stress Becomes Inflammation

The process through which psychological stress produces physical inflammation remains unclear. A major study was published that explains this process thoroughly.

Scientists conducted laboratory stress tests on healthy participants. They observed specific activation in 17 of 19 volunteers while their catecholamines and cortisol levels increased immediately after stress exposure before returning to normal levels in 60 minutes. This factor functions as a cellular switch that activates inflammatory processes.

According to the study, noradrenaline (norepinephrine) acts as a primary stress hormone that triggers inflammatory mechanisms in immune cells. The biological process transforms psychological distress into inflammatory cell responses, which occur in just minutes.

The Vicious Cycle

After inflammation enters the brain system, it generates an endless cycle of inflammation. The brain contains microglia, which act as immune cells that receive activation signals from inflammatory signals. The protective housekeeping function of these cells transforms into destructive behavior when exposed to prolonged inflammation, which leads them to produce more inflammatory substances.

The research term "inflammatory soup" describes how the mixture of inflammatory factors damages brain cells while making it harder for the brain to remove proteins, which contribute to mental decline. The described mechanism reveals why long-term inflammation elevates the chances of developing depression and dementia.

Practical Steps to Cool the Flames

Evidence-based methods exist to combat chronic inflammation and promote mental health support:

1. *Embrace Anti-Inflammatory Foods*

The Mediterranean diet stands as one of the most extensively studied dietary patterns for its anti-inflammatory effects. Focus on:

The diet should comprise abundant amounts of fruits and vegetables, which are rich in antioxidants, whole grains, legumes, and fatty fish like salmon and sardines that are rich in omega-3 fatty acids. Additionally, olive oil should be the primary fat source, and nuts and seeds should be included, with a minimal consumption of processed foods and red meat.

2. *Feed Your Good Bacteria*

Your gut microbiome acts as a central element in both inflammation processes and mood regulation. Beneficial bacteria need support through the following actions:

The diet should include fermented foods such as yogurt, kefir, sauerkraut, and kimchi.

Use antibiotics only in situations where their use is absolutely required. You don't want to kill the good bacteria along with the bad, and that's what you're doing here if you use antibiotics casually. You should consult your healthcare provider before taking any probiotic supplement because you need a high-quality product.

3. *Move Your Body Regularly*

How often have we read that exercise is one of the most important ways to manage both stress and mental health issues? But how many health care professionals indicate exercise in their treatment plans? Who gets a prescription to join a gym for exercise, and if they did, how much better would they be?

Regular moderate exercise stands as the most potent anti-inflammatory intervention available, even though intense exercise temporarily causes inflammation. Physical exercise reduces persistent inflammation, according to research, and being inactive is associated with persistent systemic inflammation.

The recommended weekly amount can be achieved through activities including brisk walking, swimming, cycling, dancing, yoga, or tai chi.

4. *Prioritize Sleep Quality*

The process of inflammation exists both as a cause and an effect of insufficient sleep. You should create a sleep-conducive environment through these steps:

The bedroom environment should be kept cool in temperature, dark, and quiet. A regular evening schedule should be followed as part of your bedtime routine.

You should refrain from using screens for an hour before bedtime. Caffeine consumption should be limited to the time before 2 PM.

5. *Manage Stress Effectively*

Stress management techniques need development because psychological stress directly causes inflammation, according to research.

Daily mindfulness meditation practice of just 10 minutes will help decrease inflammatory markers.

When experiencing stress, use the 4–2–6 deep breathing method, which involves breathing in for four counts, then holding for two before exhaling for six counts.

Social support serves as a strong protective measure that reduces inflammation caused by stress.

Happiness stands as a vital factor that helps decrease stress levels, according to research.

6. *Consider Professional Help*

Seek advice from your healthcare provider regarding potential inflammation involvement in your symptoms when you experience ongoing mood issues, particularly with inflammatory conditions.

The discussion should include whether inflammation contributes to your symptoms.

The Future of Mental Health Treatment

The modern era brings opportunities for highly customized treatments in mental health care. Research shows that depression has inflammation as its main cause in approximately 1 out of 4 patients according to recent studies.

The scientific community is currently developing three new treatments for these patients:

• Anti-inflammatory medications traditionally used for arthritis

The semaglutide GLP-1 drug shows anti-inflammatory properties among its therapeutic benefits

• Targeted therapies based on individual inflammatory profiles

• Personalized nutrition and lifestyle interventions

A New Understanding of Mental Health

The scientific breakthrough in studying inflammation and mental health functions as a transformative method for understanding depression and anxiety. A combination of biological origins from lifestyle changes and medical interventions points to more effective treatment of these psychological conditions.

Therapy and social support, along with traditional methods, remain essential. The identification of inflammation through diet, exercise, stress management, and sometimes medication becomes necessary for many patients who seek recovery.

Moving Forward

The recommended lifestyle modifications work for everyone, so you can start with these first. But don't hesitate to seek professional help if you're struggling. A healthcare provider who understands the inflammation-mental health connection can help determine if this perspective might be useful in your specific situation.

Understanding the biological elements of mental health does not decrease their complexity but provides additional methods to enhance your well-being. The development of mental health results from multiple biological factors that combine with psychological elements and social interactions. Taking care of inflammation represents an essential step in solving one part of the complex puzzle.

Chapter 67: Pain Perception May Be Related to Your Eye Coloring

Look in the mirror. What color are your eyes? Brown? Blue? Green? Does it matter about anything other than how good you think you look or what other people think you look like?

Eye coloring has a particular attraction, and that's what drove the market for colored contact lenses, where people could change from brown to green to blue or even purple or wilder eye designs. Of course, you've seen the entertainer Marilyn Manson and what he's done to his eyes.

What you see staring back at you in the mirror might hold clues about how much pain you can handle — and it's not your imagination. They say the eyes are the mirrors of the soul, but they may also indicate something else — something you may never have realized and that science is discovering.

Scientists have been quietly studying something that sounds almost too strange to be true: your eye color may predict how sensitive you are to pain. This isn't some folk tale anyone passed down to you. Today, researchers at major universities have been investigating this connection for over a decade, and their findings could change how doctors treat pain in the future. This would be a very good start to improving pain treatment for many individuals who have been discriminated against in this care.

Why Your Eyes Matter More Than You Think

Most of us think our eye color is just a random trait we inherited from our parents — nice to look at, but not particularly important. But your eyes are actually windows into your body's pain-processing system.

The key player in this story is something called melanin. You've probably heard of melanin before — it's the same stuff that determines your skin color and how easily you tan. But melanin does much more than protect you from sunburn. The same genetic pathways that control melanin production in your eyes also influence how your nervous system handles pain signals.

Now that they're finding that in research, it seems so simple to add it to the considerations for pain management. But are they doing that? Is everybody keeping up on this research? It should cause concern for all of us if they aren't.

People with brown eyes have lots of melanin packed into their irises. Those with blue or green eyes have much less. And this difference might explain why some people wince at a paper cut while others barely flinch during medical procedures. I've been an unfortunate bystander when I heard a healthcare professional express a belief that people of color didn't need as much pain medication, "because they don't feel pain the way we do."

I wasn't sure if that was correct because I didn't have the science to know. Now, I am reminded of some of those horrific slave photographs in the Harvard Peabody Museum.

What the Research Actually Shows

Dr. Inna Belfer from the University of Pittsburgh has been leading some of the most interesting work in this area. Her team studied women during childbirth — one of the most intense pain experiences humans face. What they discovered was eye-opening: women with dark brown or hazel eyes showed more signs of distress during labor than women with light-colored eyes.

The dark-eyed women didn't just experience more pain during the actual delivery. They also had more trouble sleeping because of pain, felt more discomfort when resting, and were more likely to develop depression related to their pain experience.

But there's a twist to this story. Those same dark-eyed individuals often respond better to pain medications. Their nervous systems are more reactive, which means they feel pain more intensely, but they also get more dramatic relief from treatments that work.

I recall standing in a patient's room in a hospital where a Hispanic woman had a hysterectomy and was asking the female gynecologist for more pain relief. The gynecologist refused and told her she was being discharged. I couldn't understand why she wouldn't give her more pain medication when there was a drip available that could have been made ready for her. To me, it reeked of bias. But I had no say in the matter because I was visiting a friend, another patient.

A 2024 study published in Pain Research and Management looked at women having dental work. The researchers found that eye color affected both how much pain the women felt and how well the anesthesia worked. While the results are still being debated, the pattern keeps showing up: physical characteristics like eye color seem to influence our pain experience.

The Science Behind the Connection

So what's actually happening in your body? It all comes down to genetics and brain chemistry.

The genes that produce melanin are part of a complex system that also affects your nervous system. When you have more melanin (and darker eyes), certain chemical messengers in your brain work differently. These neurotransmitters control how pain signals travel from your body to your brain.

Think of it like this: if pain signals are cars driving on a highway to your brain, people with different eye colors have different speed limits on their highways. Some people's pain signals cruise along slowly, while others race to the brain at top speed.

Recent research has uncovered even more specific mechanisms. Scientists at Massachusetts General Hospital found that the same receptor that determines red hair color — the melanocortin-1 receptor — also affects pain sensitivity. When this receptor doesn't work properly (as in people with red hair), it changes the balance of natural pain-blocking and pain-enhancing chemicals in the body. The term 'flaming red hair' may indicate more than we thought.

What This Means for Different Eye Colors

Brown Eyes: The Sensitive Responders People with brown or hazel eyes tend to be more sensitive to pain, but this isn't necessarily a bad thing. Research shows they often respond better to pain medications. Their nervous systems are more reactive, which means they feel pain more intensely, but they also respond more dramatically to treatments.

Light Eyes: The Natural Pain Blockers People with blue, green, or light-colored eyes seem to have built-in biological pain tolerance. The lower melanin levels in their eyes, according to research, correlate with brain chemistry that naturally dampens pain signals. A 2017 study found that people with dark eyes and hair showed higher pain sensitivity when their hands were placed in ice water compared to those with light features.

Red Hair: A Special Case Redheads are in a category of their own. Multiple studies have shown they're more resistant to certain types of anesthesia and may need higher doses of pain medication for some procedures. But who thinks of this? Are anesthesiologists sufficiently trained to notice this? Yet they also seem to have higher pain thresholds for certain types of pain stimuli. One of my grandmothers had incredibly red hair until the day she died in her early 50s. I hadn't been born yet, but I wonder how she was treated in the hospital for her pain.

The Real-World Impact

This research goes beyond academic curiosity. Understanding the connection between physical traits and pain could revolutionize medical practice. Imagine walking into a doctor's office where your eye color helps predict how you'll respond to different pain treatments.

Think of how normal it would be to receive adequate pain medication and not have to feel like you need to plead for it. Some patients, indeed, have to beg for it, and then they are seen as medication-seeking. I recall one man with a particular birth defect in his spine (spina bifida) who requires pain medication. He was always having to go hat-in-hand to his specialist, who reluctantly gave him less medication than he needed. The man now advocates for pain medication for those with specific medical needs. I wonder how well he will treat this research, and I hope he sees it.

Some dentists are already paying attention to this research. The 2024 dental study showed that eye color affected both pain perception and healing time after procedures. While the findings are still being studied, healthcare providers are beginning to recognize that visible characteristics might play a role in personalized pain management.

The Bigger Picture and Important Limitations

Of course, eye color isn't the only thing that affects how you experience pain. Your age, gender, overall health, stress levels, cultural background, and life experiences all play important roles. Eye color is just one piece of a much larger, more complex puzzle.

It's also crucial to understand the limitations of this research. Most studies have been small, often focusing on specific populations like women during childbirth or dental patients. The science isn't settled yet, and there's more work to be done. But we now have something to look into more intensively in terms of pain management.

Research Biases We Need to Address

This field of research has some important biases that affect how we should interpret the findings:

Limited Demographics: Most studies have focused primarily on women and people of European descent. We don't know if these patterns hold true across all racial and ethnic groups.

Small Sample Sizes: Many studies have included fewer than 100 participants, which makes it difficult to draw broad conclusions. In other words, what we call the universe of patients is still awaiting results from larger, multi-year studies.

Cultural and Social Factors: Pain expression varies significantly across cultures, but this research hasn't adequately accounted for these differences. In some cultures, it's not acceptable to admit to having pain; therefore, we don't know how research studies there would fare.

Systemic Healthcare Bias: Research has shown that medical professionals often treat pain differently based on patients' race and gender, which could skew study results. Consider how many women are seen as anxious when what they are experiencing is an actual, painful condition. Recall the woman who had the gynecologic surgery I mentioned earlier in this article.

Publication Bias: Studies showing connections are more likely to be published than those showing no relationship, which might make the evidence seem stronger than it actually is.

Researchers are often captives of the "publish or perish" mentality and funding that is aimed at proving something, such as a medication's efficacy. How many professional publications publish studies that disprove a medication or find nothing? I know a healthcare professional who discovered something that didn't make it to publication, but it earned him a patent that made him a millionaire.

Looking Forward

As genetic testing becomes more common and affordable, we're likely to see much more research connecting physical traits to health outcomes. Your eye color might just be the tip of the iceberg. Scientists are currently studying how pigmentation affects drug metabolism, disease risk, and other biological processes.

One thing is clear: our physical characteristics have a more complex and fascinating relationship with our internal experiences than we previously thought. Your eye color might be providing biological information that could lead to better, more personalized medical care in the future.

While we wait for more research to confirm and build upon these findings, it's exciting to think that something as simple as eye color could someday help doctors provide better pain relief for everyone, especially for those who need it.

Chapter 68: And Then There Was a NEW Personality "Disorder" for Pondering

Have you ever sat in a room full of friends, coworkers, or family members and felt completely alone? Not because they weren't nice to you,but because something deep inside you just couldn't connect with the group energy? If you've always been the person who skips the team-building exercises, avoids group vacations, and prefers one-on-one conversations over parties, you might be what psychiatrist Dr. Rami Kaminski calls an "otrovert."

After 40 years of treating patients, Dr. Kaminski noticed something fascinating: there were people who weren't introverts or extroverts. They were something else entirely. These people could be charming and the person social, but they never felt like they truly belonged to any group — no matter how welcoming that group was. It is, however, based on his individual clinical experience.

You're Not Broken — You're Just Different

For too long, our society has only recognized two types of people: introverts (who get drained by social situations) and extroverts (who get energized by them). But both of these personality types share one crucial thing—they're what Dr. Kaminski calls "communal people." Whether they're quiet or loud, both introverts and extroverts want to be part of the group. They find safety, identity, and self-worth through their connections to others.

Otroverts are different. They're the eternal outsiders, the people who watch from the edges even when they're standing right in the center of the action. The word comes from the Spanish "otro," meaning "other"—because otroverts are always looking elsewhere, beyond the group dynamics that captivate everyone else.

Think about that friend who's incredibly likable but somehow never seems to "click" with group activities. They might be the life of the party in a one-on-one conversation, but you'll notice them checking out mentally during group discussions. That might be an otrovert.

The Science Behind Not Belonging

For decades, psychologists have studied why humans have such a powerful need to belong to groups. Social Identity Theory, developed by Henri Tajfel in the 1970s, shows that most people define themselves through their group memberships—whether it's their family, workplace, political party, or favorite sports team. This isn't just social preference; it's how our brains are wired.

Research consistently shows that when people identify with a group, they automatically start favoring that group over others.

Sounds terribly MAGA, doesn't it? The individuals adopt the group's beliefs and follow its unwritten behavior to fit in better. This "belonging instinct" has helped humans survive for thousands of years by creating strong communities and shared identities.

But otroverts seem to be missing this psychological programming. They don't get the same emotional payoff from group membership that most people do. It's not that they can't form relationships—quite the opposite. Otroverts often form incredibly deep, meaningful one-on-one relationships. They're empathetic, generous, and emotionally intelligent. They just can't seem to plug into the group matrix that most people find so natural. All of these attributes, and even the personality disorder, however, are still awaiting worldwide scientific evidence.

The Hidden Advantages of Standing Alone

Let's dig in a little deeper into this "disorder." Here's where it gets interesting: being an otrovert isn't a bug — it's a feature. When you don't belong to any group, you're free from what psychologists call "groupthink" the tendency for groups to make poor decisions because everyone goes along with the majority.

Studies on creativity and independent thinking reveal that people who resist conformity often come up with more original ideas. When you're not trying to fit in, you're not unconsciously limiting your thoughts to what the group finds acceptable. You can see problems and solutions that others miss because you're not looking through the lens of group consensus.

Research published in Cognitive Science shows that when people are exposed to ideas that challenge conventional thinking, they become more creative in their own problem-solving. Otroverts live in this space naturally — they're always outside conventional thinking because they fully buy into any group's worldview.

Some of the famous otroverts throughout history include George Orwell, who saw the dangers of political groupthink long before others; Albert Einstein, who revolutionized physics by thinking outside established scientific communities; and Franz Kafka, whose outsider perspective allowed him to capture the absurdity of modern life in ways that resonated across cultures.

How Disorders Are Included in the DSM

Although you may be thinking that you have this disorder or gift, whichever you prefer, there is one glitch here that must be considered. What is it? No one can come up with a disorder and then expect it to be put into use by persons in the healthcare professions. It doesn't happen that way. All disorders that are listed in the official "bible" of psychiatric disorders are selected and included by a committee.

The American Psychiatric Association depends on mental health expert committees to determine what will be included in the DSM (Diagnostic and Statistical Manual of Mental Disorders). Psychiatrists and researchers examine scientific research about various mental health disorders, evaluate the reliability of disorder diagnoses, and assess the potential benefits of inclusion for patient treatment improvement. If it's not in the DSM, it's not considered a psychiatric disorder. True, there is a section in the back for disorders under consideration. This might, in the future, be one of those disorders

Recognizing the Otrovert in Your Life (or Yourself

According to this new thinking on personality, introverts often fly under the radar because they've learned to mimic group behavior when necessary. They are called "pseudo-extroverts" — they can be charming and engaging in social situations, but it's a performance rather than a genuine connection to the group energy.

Here are some thoughts you might be dealing with as an introvert:

They're selective about their energy: unlike introverts, who get drained by all social interaction, otroverts can talk for hours one-on-one but seem to fade during group activities.

They resist peer pressure naturally: not because they're rebellious, but because they genuinely don't feel the social pull that makes others want to conform.

They're unusually independent thinkers: They form own opinions without being swayed by what "everyone" thinks or does. Depending on the situation, this can be a benefit or a deficit

They prefer meaningful conversations: Small talk group banter don't interest them, but they'll dive deep into topics they care about with individual people.

They're generous but not groupy: They'll go out of their way to help friends but won't join group volunteer efforts or team activities.

Thriving as an Otrovert in a Group-Obsessed World

If you recognize yourself in this description, there's nothing wrong with you, but don't use this as a reason for everything that you do. Remember, it's still someone's interesting idea about personality.

Society tells us that we need to be team players, join communities, and find our tribe. But otroverts have a different path to fulfillment.

The key is understanding that your need for independence isn't antisocial —it's how you function best. Instead of forcing yourself into group situations that drain you, focus on building those deep one-on-one relationships where you shine.

In the workplace, otroverts often excel in roles that require independent thinking: research, writing, consulting, or any position where original ideas are valued over group consensus. They make excellent advisors because they're not invested in any particular outcome except finding the truth. To me, this smacks of a type of autism. Aren't many of these characteristics similar to it?

Parents of otrovert children should resist the urge to push them into group activities. Instead, encourage one-on-one friendships and give them space to pursue their individual interests without pressure to "join in."

The Gift of Perspective

In our increasingly polarized world, otroverts offer something valuable: the ability to see beyond tribal thinking. While others get caught up in "us versus them" mentalities, otroverts can maintain perspective because they never fully identify with any "us" in the first place. But, seemingly, it's not a lonely place.

Research on conformity shows that having even one person who thinks independently can dramatically improve group decision-making. It's critical thinking comes into play, and I have written an entire book on it (The Little Book on Learning Big Critical Thinking Skills) that is being published. When everyone else is nodding along, the otrovert in the room might be the only one asking the difficult questions that lead to better outcomes.

Embracing Your Authentic Self

The message for otroverts is simple: stop trying to fix something that isn't broken. Your inability to "belong" isn't a character flaw — it's a different way of being human that comes with its own gifts.

For those who love an otrovert, the best thing you can do is accept them as they are. Don't try to pull them into group activities; they're clearly uncomfortable with them. Instead, value the unique perspective they bring and the depth of relationship they can offer when it's just the two of you.

Otroverts are like, as Dr. Rami Kaminski said, "Bluetooth devices that just aren't wired for group pairing." They connect differently, but when they do connect, it's often deeper and more meaningful than the connections most people experience in groups.

In a world that constantly pushes us to join, belong, and conform, otroverts remind us that there's another way to live —authentically, independently, and with the kind of perspective that can only come from standing slightly outside the crowd.

Chapter 69: The Height Problem No One Wants to Talk About

As you enter a job interview, you discover through instinct that the interviewer has already formed impressions about your leadership potential based solely on your height. Somehow this doesn't seem reasonable. And it's not paranoia or overthinking. The bias affects millions of people every day yet people avoid discussing it openly.

Statistics confirm that being short results in actual monetary losses. Studies in the Journal of Applied Psychology demonstrated that male workers earn higher wages by about 2 percent for each extra inch of height. A 6-foot-tall man earns more money than his 5'6" counterpart annually due to height differences without any impact on their intelligence skills or work ethic.

The Hidden Discrimination in Plain Sight

Height discrimination also known as "heightism" stands as one of the least discussed prejudices in our contemporary society. The available data indicates that ninety percent of CEOs possess above-average height measurements and only three percent have heights below 5'7". The acceptance of height-based leadership limitations continues despite our modern push for diversity and anti-discrimination practices. Why such an emphasis on height? Maybe it's because instinctively it is associated with a number of urban myths or even evolutionary myths.

Our ordinary language perpetuates this discriminatory pattern. People who impress us physically stand above us while people we dismiss physically stand below us. People praise someone's "towering intellect" and describe respected individuals as having "impressive stature." When shorter individuals demonstrate powerful opinions people usually label them as having "Napoleon complex" while tall individuals show the same confidence without receiving such judgment.

Dr. Tanya Osensky who stands at 4'11" documented these personal experiences through her research on height discrimination. Her research demonstrates that people reject discriminatory attitudes toward short individuals because heightism continues to remain an unacknowledged legitimate discriminatory practice.

A Journey Through History's Beauty Standards

The fixation on height has existed since ancient times but its intensity has never reached current levels. Throughout time beauty standards have transformed like shifting desert dunes. In ancient Greece, the perfect woman was characterized by her plump figure combined with wide hips and small breasts. The Renaissance era brought about a beauty standard which included large forehead sizes so women would shave their hairlines to create an appearance of greater forehead dimensions.

The 1700s and early 1800s emphasized physical balance because beauty standards required women to maintain proportions between their height and other body measurements. The cultural focus during this time centered on moderation rather than extremes. During medieval times, women who carried extra weight were considered attractive because it signified wealth while skinny women were linked to poverty or religious devotion.

During the 17th century, the Sun King, Louis XIV of France, who reigned for 72 years in France, earned his nickname "Le Talon Rouge" because he wore red-heeled shoes, which became the ultimate symbol of status and privilege across Europe. Today, of course, we have the uber-rich wearing red-soled shoes, Louboutin.

He mandated red-heeled footwear for anyone wishing to enter his luxurious Versailles court. Only nobles had the right to wear red heels, with their social status determining the maximum height of their heels. Louis XIV often wore heels that reached four inches, which heightened his already commanding presence.

These fashion choices served as tools for political influence. Don't we still see certain expensive items as portraying importance and influence? The expensive red dye and impractical shoes indicated that the wearer possessed enough wealth to avoid both walking on dirt and performing manual labor. The sight of crimson heels gliding across marble floors signaled that authentic power was approaching. We're not talking about ballet here when we say "The Red Shoes."

The fashion trend expanded throughout Europe yet Louis XIV maintained his position as the most influential trendsetter who demonstrated that minor details reveal the most about true authority. I don't know about you, but red-soled shoes seem highly impractical unless you never have to walk anywhere.

I wonder how my local shoemaker would have handled re-soleing those shoes. He re-soled plenty of my shoes when I was in elementary school. In fact, he re-soled them so often, they were like rockers on the bottom of my shoes. There is only so many times you can half-sole a child's oxford.

Western society at some point established an unprecedented connection between height and power as well as success and attractiveness that previous civilizations never established. The belief in male stature superiority emerged from 19th century eugenic and Social Darwinist movements which developed pseudoscientific theories about tall men being superior.

The Psychological Impact of Being Short

The consequences of height discrimination extend well past financial losses. Research showed that height satisfaction rates were extremely low among short men reaching only 26% but very high among tall men at 87%. The enormous height satisfaction difference between tall and short men shows how deeply our height-obsessed culture affects their mental state. The more it appears that height is a definite advantage in dating.

Research conducted with Swedish men established that social class directly linked to height while showing height increases resulted in lower suicide rates. The combination of short stature and lower social standing made men more prone to suicidal thoughts which highlights the fatal nature of height discrimination.

Chinese research revealed that men who were unhappy with their height displayed avoidance behaviors when encountering height-related words which demonstrates how deep their psychological distress has become.

When Desperation Leads to Drastic Measures

People, seemingly men in particular, who experience severe height discrimination may choose to undergo dangerous surgical procedures to achieve minimal height growth. They are now choosing to undergo leg-lengthening surgery which costs $75,000 while requiring doctors to break their bones and stretch them apart over several months.

Doctors perform this procedure by placing telescopic rods into fractured bones and using external remote controls to extend them at 1 millimeter per day for two to three months. The medical procedure requires patients to remain bedridden for weeks and carries risks of infection alongside potential nerve damage and joint complications.

According to research it has been revealed that one in ten young men between 16 and 24 years of age considered undergoing leg-lengthening surgery. It would seem a rather drastic way to handle something that may not be related to height. For example, look at some of the world leaders and their stature. Leader of the Ukraine, Volodymyr Zelenskyy is 5 feet 7 inches, while Ireland's Michael D. Higgins is 5 feet, 3 inches, UK Prime Minister Rishi Sunak is 5 feet, 6 inches, and France's Emmanuel Macron is 5 feet, 7 inches.

The goal of some of these leg-lengthening procedures is to grow from 5 feet 7 inches to 6 feet and an ultimate goal of reaching 6 feet 2 inches. According to one patient, his depression stemmed from his height while he acknowledged that undergoing the "very painful, very hard" procedure led him to believe his new height would help him "reach everything in life." The sad fact is, it may have nothing to do with his height at all.

The Professional Price of Being Short

Height bias at work generates specific measurable consequences that have substantial impact. Research shows that taller men and women receive more leader-like perceptions from others while being perceived as intelligent and healthy than their shorter colleagues. The recruitment process favors taller candidates because recruiters consider them more skilled and employable. Then, of course, there is "the beauty effect." There is even a scale to determine who is more culturally acceptable as beautiful and who is not. I Out the validity of the scales since it was on a very small sample in Nepal. But beauty does get people certain advantages, and the beauty market will prosper as a result.

The Chinese government has outlawed height requirements for employment yet certain positions including bank staff and lawyers and airline personnel must have a minimum height of 5 feet 7 inches. Research in China during a ten-year period demonstrated that employees with shorter stature earned reduced wages than taller employees who held similar positions.

Breaking the Height Ceiling

Society faces a significant political and social challenge because of income loss caused by short stature particularly when short stature emerges from childhood poverty and malnutrition plus the effects of ADHD medications. However, there is a bit of blowback on the latter. According to research well-nourished and healthy childhood development leads to both physical and cognitive success.

The process repeats itself when economically disadvantaged children fail to achieve their complete height because of inadequate nutrition leading to height-based discrimination in adulthood, which maintains social inequality.

Standing Up for Change

Surgery or accepting discrimination do not provide the solution because we need to transform how society views height in relation to leadership. It seems that we have already crossed that bridge in international politics. Employers now understand that remote work can help decrease height bias since height cannot be easily assessed through video conferencing.

But real change requires more than corporate policies. Each person needs to analyze their own prejudice. When you unconsciously believe taller people have more capability and shorter people have less authority, take a moment to evaluate if your judgment is based on genetic makeup.

Height discrimination survives through the lack of open discussion. The first step toward building an equitable society begins with open dialogue about height bias because we should judge people based on their character and contributions rather than their physical height.

Throughout history, influential figures such as Napoleon, Martin Luther King Jr. and Mother Teresa demonstrated that true stature exists beyond physical height because their impact on the world determined their actual size. I wonder how tall Jesus was.

Chapter 70: Surprise! Your Aging Brain Isn't Wearing Thin — It's Retrofitting Its Layers

Most of us have heard the same warning about getting older: the brain gradually shrinks, nerve cells are lost, and mental sharpness fades. It's a neat, simple story—but it isn't quite true. Groundbreaking research in Nature Neuroscience suggests something far more dynamic is happening inside the aging brain. Instead of a uniform, across-the-board decline, the brain appears to remodel itself with remarkable precision — layer by layer. This discovery challenges long-standing assumptions and opens the door to a new way of thinking about brain aging.

The brain's outer layer, the cerebral cortex, is arranged a bit like a multi-tiered cake, each horizontal sheet with its own role. Middle layer IV receives and processes incoming sensory information — everything you feel, see, and hear starts here. The deeper layers send necessary output signals to other brain areas and help regulate the delicate balance between excitation and inhibition.

The outermost layers link nearby areas together, coordinating complex networks. For many years, it was assumed these layers aged in roughly the same way, with generalized thinning and loss. But when scientists looked closer, they found the story was more complicated. One group that has begun to be studied is the super agers. The results indicate that there is hope, not despair, that comes with new aging research.

Using ultra-high-resolution MRI in humans and imaging in mice, researchers mapped these cortical layers in exquisite detail. The results were surprising. In older adults, the middle layer was thicker and more heavily myelinated — the process by which nerve fibers are insulated with fatty sheaths to speed transmission — compared with younger adults.

The deeper layers, responsible for output and modulation, were indeed thinner with age, but they too showed an increase in myelination. Outer layers changed very little. This is not the pattern you'd expect if aging were simply erosion. It's a patchwork of loss and reinforcement, as if the brain is strategically shoring up specific circuits while letting others shrink. We have to wonder if this process is related to learning and intense cognition; it may be, and also lifestyle. Why else would the brain be doing this? We know exercise affects mood as well as hormone deliveries, and now maybe exercise does more than that. It sends a signal deep within the brain to initiate this restorative and reinforcing function.

What's the Reason?

Why would the input layer expand and gain more insulation? One possibility is compensation. As we age, the receptors in our skin and other sense organs become less sensitive; signals arriving from the outside world grow weaker. By thickening and myelinating the neurons in the layer that handles incoming information, the brain may be increasing the "volume" to ensure messages still get through. It's almost like the brain's hearing aid has been turned up.

In essence, it's boosting the volume on a fuzzy microphone. The deeper layers are a puzzle of their own. Even as they lose tissue, they gain insulation. Might this be an active process to keep the delicate electrical signals from slipping away through the membrane? This may reflect an effort to keep their long-distance communication stable despite having fewer cells. In other words, the brain might be reinforcing specific control circuits to maintain stability in the system. This is more than amazing. And we don't know if there is a master portion of the brain that has control over all of it

These insights fit with what other research tells us about myelin throughout life. Myelination doesn't peak in childhood and then simply fade; it moves in waves. Some regions gain more insulation well into middle age, while others decline earlier or later. Certain conditions trigger increases in myelination as a form of adaptation. Like muscles responding to training, the brain's layers seem capable of bulking up or trimming down depending on what's needed. But how is the need determined, and what mechanism is behind it?

The Effect of Neurologic Illness

The idea of targeted remodeling also has medical implications. Different brain diseases affect different layers in different ways. Multiple sclerosis often damages specific cortical layers, disrupting communication between regions. Alzheimer's typically begins in superficial layers before reaching deeper circuits. Knowing exactly which layers adapt and which ones are vulnerable could help doctors design precision therapies, from medication to noninvasive brain stimulation, aimed at protecting or enhancing the right circuits at the right time.

Experience may also play a role. Animal studies have shown that learning certain skills can change the thickness and connectivity of particular layers, while sensory deprivation can cause them to shrink. This means the changes we see in aging brains may not be purely the result of time alone. They could be shaped by a lifetime of habits, environments, and activities. A person who has worked with fine tactile details — like a weaver or a pianist — might preserve or even enhance certain features well into old age.

If that's true, the usual advice for "keeping your brain young" might need a twist. Activities that broadly stimulate the mind, like learning a language, playing chess, or solving puzzles, are still beneficial, but we might eventually design lifestyle routines that specifically target particular layers.

One layer could be strengthened through rich sensory input: crafts, texture-based games, or skillful handwork that demands fine touch. While such "layer-specific brain training" is still speculative, it's a logical extension of these findings. Now, of course, the challenge is to find activities that will produce the changes we seek in specific individuals

Seen in this light, the aging brain isn't simply in retreat. Can you think of better news for people who are aging? And, of course, everyone is aging. Our brains are now seen as actively re-engineering themselves, making choices about where to invest their resources. Some of those choices may be compensatory, keeping us functioning despite losses elsewhere. Others may set the stage for resilience. This research suggests that even late in life, the brain has options — it's not passively succumbing to entropy.

This is why reframing brain aging matters. We've often heard the term "reframing" in psychotherapy and even in critical thinking. Still, we need to consider this in terms of our brains. If we can think of it less as a slow slide and more as a remodeling project, we can start looking for ways to work with those changes instead of against them. It also invites a more hopeful perspective. In a society where people are living longer, we need to begin to look at age in a different way and through a different lens.

The truth is, our brains may not be wearing thin after all. They may be rewiring themselves to keep us connected, responsive, and adaptable for as long as possible. Recognizing this could be the first step toward designing lives, therapies, and public health strategies that help the brain use this remarkable flexibility to our advantage. After all, we are in an age where AI has incredible abilities to come up with strategies that may benefit the brain's resilience and the people whose heads they reside in. Let's begin to use that technology in this area.

About the Author

D
r. Patricia A. Farrell is a licensed psychologist, published author of multiple self-help books and videos, former WebMD psychologist expert/consultant, medical consultant for Social Security Disability Determinations, Alzheimer's psychiatric researcher at Mt. Sinai Medical Center (NYC), and an educator who has taught at the college, graduate, and postgraduate levels.

Her influence extends to the pharmaceutical and marketing industries, where she serves as a consultant and has appeared on major TV news programs in the US and abroad. In addition, Dr. Farrell provides continuing education modules for mental healthcare professionals and has contributed to USMLE medical school prep courses. She shares her knowledge through her YouTube channel and her daily contributions to **Bluesky** (@carpenter22,bsky.social) and Medium. com articles. Dr. Farrell's achievements are recognized in *Who's Who in the World, Who's Who in America,* and *Who's Who in American Women.*

A member of the American Psychological Association and the SAG-AFTRA union, Dr. Farrell is a former board member of the NJ Board of Psychological Examiners, a former psychiatry preceptor at UMDNJ, and a former board of directors member of Bergen Pines Hospital (now Bergen Regional Hospital).

Books by Patricia A. Farrell, Ph.D.

How to Be Your Own Therapist

When You Can't Pour From an Empty Glass: CBT Skills for Exhausted Caregivers

The Little Book on Learning Big Critical Thinking Skills

It's Not All in Your Head: Anxiety, Depression, Mood Swings and Multiple Sclerosis

Unfiltered: Beneath the noise of our thoughts lies the true narrative of our minds

Unfiltered Again: A behind-the-scenes look at healthcare, medicine and mental health

When You Can't Pour From an Empty Glass: CBT Skills for Exhausted Caregivers

A Social Security Disability Psychological Claims Handbook: A simple guide to understanding your SSD claim for psychological impairments and unraveling the maze of decision-making

A Social Security Disability Psychological Claims Guidebook for Children's Benefits

The Disability Accessible US Parks in All 50 States: A Comprehensive Guide

Birding in the US NOW!: A birding guide for individuals with disabilities

Books by Dr. Patricia A. Farrell

How to Be Your Own Therapist

    The Little Book on Learning Big Critical Thinking Skills

When You Can't Pour From an Empty Glass: CBT Skills for Exhausted Caregivers

It's Not All in Your Head: Anxiety, Depression, Mood Swings and Multiple Sclerosis

Unfiltered: Beneath the noise of our thoughts lies the true narrative of our minds

Unfiltered Again: A behind-the-scenes look at healthcare, medicine and mental health

Unfiltered Redux: Exploring uncharted depths of mind where masks fall and wisdom emerges

A Social Security Disability Psychological Claims Handbook: A simple guide to understanding your SSD claim for psychological impairments and unraveling the maze of decision-making

A Social Security Disability Psychological Claims Guidebook for Children's Benefits

The Disability Accessible US Parks in All 50 States: A Comprehensive Guide

Birding in the US NOW!: A birding guide for individuals with disabilities

A Special Request

I f this book has touched your heart, sparked your curiosity, or simply entertained you along the way, I'd be incredibly grateful if you could take a moment to share your thoughts with a review on Amazon or wherever you discovered this book. Your words not only help other readers find books they'll love, but they also mean the world to authors like me who pour their hearts into every page. Thank you for being part of this journey, and for helping stories find their way to the readers who need them most.